THE WWII BOMBING OF BARI, ITALY

The WWII Bombing of Bari, Italy
Copyright © 2025 Vincent dePaul Lupiano

All rights reserved under the Pan-American and International Copyright Conventions. This book may not be reproduced in whole or in part, except for brief quotations embodied in critical articles or reviews, in any form or by any means, electronic or mechanical, including photocopying, recording, or by any information storage and retrieval system now known or hereinafter invented, without written permission of the publisher.

This book is based on the author's research, experiences, and opinions. While every effort has been made to ensure accuracy, the author and publisher make no representations or warranties about the completeness, reliability, or applicability of the content. This book is for informational purposes only and should not be considered professional advice. The author and publisher assume no liability for any actions taken based on the information presented.

ISBN Paperback: 978-1-963271-92-8
ISBN Ebook: 978-1-963271-93-5

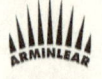

Published by Armin Lear Press, Inc.
215 W Riverside Drive, #4362
Estes Park, CO 80517

THE WWII BOMBING OF BARI, ITALY

THE CLASSIFIED DISASTER AND COVERUP THAT LAUNCHED THE DISCOVERY OF CHEMOTHERAPY

VINCENT dePAUL LUPIANO

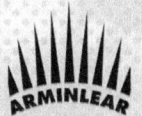
ARMINLEAR

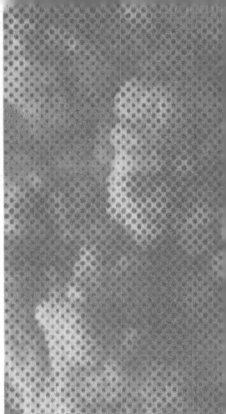

AUTHOR'S NOTE

While this book includes a comprehensive bibliography of the principal sources consulted during the research and writing process, many other works—books, periodicals, archival materials, and firsthand accounts—also contributed to my understanding of the events described. These additional references provided valuable context and insight, even if they are not cited directly. I am deeply indebted to the many historians, journalists, scholars, and eyewitnesses whose work has helped illuminate this remarkable chapter of history.

Specifically, many thanks to the following:

Contance Pechura's and David Raoul's *Veterans at Risk: The Health Effects of Mustard Gas*;

Vincent Orange, a biography of Air Marshal Sir Arthur Coningham; D.M. Saunders', "The Bari Incident."

Multiple sources for details regarding the bombing of Dresden, Germany.

From History.com, *How a WWII Disaster—and Cover-up—Led to a Cancer Treatment Breakthrough.*

From Smithsonian Magazine: *The Bombing and the Breakthrough: How A Chemical Weapons Disaster In World War II Led To A U.S. Cover-Up—And A New Cancer Treatment.*

CONTENTS

1	The Hag	1
2	Liberty Ships	21
3	Henry Cronbach Lowenhaupt	35
4	"The Swedish Turnip"	49
5	General James Harold "Jimmy" Doolittle	69
6	The Devil In Mufti	75
7	A Welter of Surprise	85
8	"Che cosa?"	91
9	"I smell garlic."	103
10	The Devil's Doing	119
11	Burns–"Not Yet Determined"	137
12	The Father of Chemotherapy	151
13	Bari	159
Coda		175
Bibliography		183
About the Author		185

*To the men and women who suffered
and gave their lives on 2 Dec. 1943*

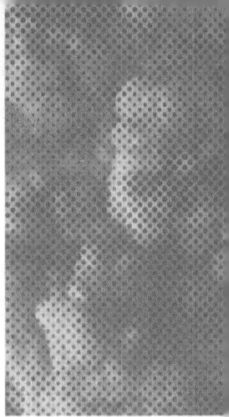

1

THE HAG

2 Dec. 1943 - 1105 hours - Grosseto Main Airport, Italy – Few people know the extent of what happened at Bari, Italy, on 2 Dec. 1943. Until now.

* * *

Luftwaffe *Hauptmann* (Captain) Veit Renz climbs into the cockpit of a careworn Messerschmitt Me 210 fighter bomber at the end of the dispersal area. In seventy-eight minutes, the *Hauptmann* will be fast-moving through 23,000 feet in a pilot's sky and flying over historic Bari, Italy—this his fifth consecutive day reconnoitering the vital port city.

When he reaches the top of the cockpit, Renz closes his eyes for a moment and shakes his head; he hates this airplane. He truly does. All the pilots, the gunners, the mechanics dislike it, too. The green-gray camouflage paint fading, lifeless.

Paused at the cockpit railing, he mutters, *"Die alt deutsche Hexe"*—the old German Hag. Shakes his head again. Summons a parcel of fighter pilot courage before he hoists his polished flying boot over the canopy rail and squeezes down into the dusty cockpit.

Design started before the war as a replacement for the Bf 110. Ready in 1939, the first Me 210 batch had unacceptably poor flight characteristics due to serious wing planform and fuselage design flaws. The design entered limited service in 1942. Some pilots said they survived a Dutch Roll—only *some*—an extremely dangerous flight maneuver named after Dutch ice skaters: side-to-side and up-and-down movement of the aircraft. Once it starts, it's almost impossible to cease oscillating.

And some pilots—more literate than most—thought the bird had "the flight characteristics of an inebriated butterfly." Some refused to strap on the aircraft because they feared it was *zu gefährlich*—too dangerous. Throughout 1941 and 1942, a large-scale operational testing program struggled for solutions but did not moderate the Hag's dubious proclivities. The failure of the Me 210's development program meant the Luftwaffe was forced to continue operating the Bf 110 after it had outlived its shelf date, despite mounting losses—only adding to the Luftwaffe's current pains throughout the Italian peninsula. The aircraft also tended to waver, even while flying level—some called it "porpoising." At first, the designers concentrated on the twin-rudder arrangement that had been copied from the 110 and replaced it with a new and much larger single vertical stabilizer that had the likeness of a shark's dorsal fin. A menacing effect but an almost zero result, and the plane continued to "snake" and remain remorseless. The Me 210 also suffered terrible stalls—one of the most difficult nightmares a pilot had to overcome, especially if he was inexperienced. With the nose up or in a turn, stalls whittled into spins, and when the aircraft spun flat, the automatic leading-edge slats opened uninvited. The chief test pilot commented that the Me 210 had "all the least desirable attributes an airplane could possess."

Nevertheless, *Hauptmann* Renz prepares to fly his fifth consecutive reconnaissance mission, leaving behind his dear Junkers 88 despite his forceful objections. The 88 helped him win his Oakleaves to the Knight's Cross and other awards pinned proudly to his flight blouse and inked with precision in his thick pilot's logbook.

Renz has done the due diligence of an *experten* pilot and has shrewdly studied Bari's harbor, again his target today: two hundred thousand or so war-weary residents residing down there in the ancient city with an intricate past—the capital of the Puglia region of Italy composed of Bari, Brindisi, and Taranto (the heel of the "boot"). Renz is mindful, too, of Bari's ancient, complicated history—one of destruction, conquest, and reconstruction. The city enjoys a warm climate and flat terrain and faces the Adriatic Sea to its west. In his heart, Renz wants to leave the beauty of Bari's architecture untouched by German bombs. Besides, he does not want to waste bombs on the city—the harbor is the target for numerous strategic reasons.

Because of its location, Bari has continuously played in a dangerous game of pawns among warring nations. The Greeks conquered Bari and its architectural splendor. Normans, Goths,

Lombards, and Saracen crusaders left their marks with swords and nefarious notions. Then, the Romans pressed in, clawed the city, and created an excellent seaport and significant center for commerce that remains today. The city's old section, a labyrinth of medieval houses, small streets, and narrow alleyways. Bari surrounded on three sides by water, and most of the houses belong primarily to fishermen earning their living on the Adriatic.

While there are several churches in Bari, the most historically important is the Basilica of San Nicola, known as Nicholas of Bari.

Because he was a secret "gift giver," San Nicola became known as *Santa Claus*, "Saint Nick" or "Father Christmas." Here in the Basilica rests his remains, stolen by sailors from Asia Minor and abandoned to spiders and cobwebs for eternity to hold.

As he had done for the previous reconnaissance flights, today Renz focuses on Bari's magnificent harbor. Shaped like a huge, irregular horseshoe with a wide aperture to the Adriatic. The harbor a perfect receptacle for Allied Liberty Ships and cargo carriers from multiple Allied countries supporting the war against Nazi Germany.

Bari has a Mediterranean climate with mild winters and hot, dry summers—today it is 56º F—and the area has always been a foremost center for shipping, today more so for its value to the Allies and their strategic intentions.

Renz, today, knows that Bari can be the most important target so far in the entire Italian peninsula, the whole campaign—in fact, in all of Europe, with the potential for effecting the outcome of WWII. He thinks of Italy as a great path for the Germans to march up from the south, from Sicily, from Bari, all the way up into Europe, Germany specifically, and tear the war to their advantage. The importance of the harbor and his mission had given him a sense of abundant pride. This sort of ameliorates his negative attitude toward the Me 210 that he is sliding down into.

Bright December sun has baked the metal cockpit for the past four hours, and now the seat, the controls, the canopy rails are as hot as a griddle. Squeezing into his gloves, Veit checks his Hanhart wristwatch. Below him, *Feldwebel* (Staff Sergeant) Hurdelbrink has his plump face inside the number one Daimler-Benz engine bay.

"*Was machst du?*" Veit asks the crew chief.

"*Sie braucht einen Liter Öl!*"

Renz mutters "*Scheiße!*" Shit. Examines a smudge of cloud against a delicate blue sky for an answer. Rolls his eyes: *now you are telling me this piece of cow shit needs oil—minutes before I take off?*

"*Tut mir leid,*" says Hurdelbrink, apologizing.

Veit tells the crew chief that there must be a small oil leak somewhere because reliable engines like the Daimler Benz DB don't just lose a quart of oil in the time this bird's been sitting here. So now the *Hauptmann* has to fly the Hag over two hours to and from Bari with a possible oil leak that could develop into a catastrophe.

He's pissed.

"*Scheiße!*" he says again to the gas gauges that are not listening to him.

Then looking down at Hurdelbrink, "*Mir läuft die Zeit davon.*" This will put me behind the flight plan, he tells the crew chief.

When Veit returns from the reconnaissance mission, he will

have a chat with Hurdelbrink's maintenance officer about the oil problem. Little good it will do; there's barely a drop to spare these days. The situation here in Italy, throughout the Luftwaffe, is dire and complex, and there are more impactful problems than small oil leaks. But small or not, an oil leak could lose a battle—a war! The toll on German planes and pilots has been mainly because support from the Italian Air Force is practically nonexistent. And the Allied supplies pouring into Italy right now at Bari appear endless and need to be stopped immediately.

Squeezing into the pilot's seat, scorching his butt. The cockpit smelling of B4 avgas fumes and burnt engine oil. A comfort now being alone. He stows a thermos of hot, black ersatz coffee and a sandwich of thick, rustic *Baurenbrut* bread (farmer's bread) and freshly cooked *Weisswurst* sausage. He will have his lunch with the clouds and listen to the drone of his engines.

A sandpiper lands herky-jerky on the thick glinting grass off the port wingtip, scrounging for worms. One more hungry flyer on the airfield on combat patrol. The bird unscrewing a wiggler out of the turf until Hurdelbrink slams the cowling shut and replaces the pump handle and hose from the Kleintankwagen oil truck. The noise startles the sandpiper, and it flitters away from the commotion. The worm, squirming, captive in the bird's beak.

To counter the Allied army's advance and appease Adolf Hitler, *Generalfeldmsarshall* Kesselring has to restrain, diminish, or demolish General Doolittle's newly formed Fifteenth Air Force situated around Foggia—which consists of several airfields scattered about the city, too many targets for the Luftwaffe to expeditiously conduct a single strike; this presents a tactical problem. And the toll the Allies are taking on German forces and equipment is appalling, especially since the Italian Air Force is non-existent and lends trivial support to the Luftwaffe.

In keeping with his wariness of his military professionals, on 21 November 1943, Adolf Hitler let it be known that he alone had an answer to this issue, as he always did: He anointed 58-year-old *Generalfeldmarschall* (General of the Army or Field Marshal) Albert Kesselring *Oberfeldfelshaber Süd* (Commander-in-Chief South) and concurrently assigned him command of a resuscitated *Heeresguppe C* (Army Group C). Essentially, Kesselring had been elevated to supreme commander of the entire Italian peninsula for the German Army and Air Force—an officer highly regarded by Hitler for his tactical acumen. With this appointment, Hitler expected immediate results.

This was a righteous choice: Kesselring was known throughout the German army for his charismatic style of leadership. After the war and in American captivity, his American captors nicknamed him "Smilin' Al." Known to inspire and maintain the loyalty of his troops, even under challenging circumstances. His approachability and concern for the welfare of his soldiers earned him natural respect and admiration. The field marshal was highly strategic and showed great adaptability on various fronts during the war. And was skilled at managing both air and ground operations, demonstrating a keen understanding of military tactics and strategy. Kesselring had often been described as optimistic and maintaining a positive outlook even in difficult situations. It gave him the ability to look at the current dire military situation and attempt to clearly formulate a solution with ample input from his staff. This trait helped him motivate his troops and manage stress during critical military operations. Amazingly—at the age of 58, no less—the field marshal decided to take flying lessons to demonstrate unquestionable solidarity with his troops. This was an unheard-of undertaking for a man his age and position in the Luftwaffe (Hitler was not delighted when he heard about this). At age 58, the field marshal earned a pilot's license without cutting corners or "pulling rank." Plain and simple, Kesselring was not only a field marshal but now a pilot and wore a pilot's silver badge proudly on his bespoke tunic; his men were delighted. He was also a pragmatist in his approach to warfare and decisions based on practical rather than ideological considerations. Thus, he was a flexible commander who reacted dynamically to the realities of the battlefield. These traits contributed to his effectiveness as a military leader and were key to his success in coordinating extensive military campaigns across various European theaters. His personality and leadership style were significant factors in his ability to maintain cohesion and morale among his forces during critical phases of the war.

Today, Kesselring and staff are headquartered at Frascati, twenty-one kilometers southwest of Rome—until 8 September 1943 when it was bombed; then, they moved to Monte Soratte. The mountain played an important role for the Germans during World War II—it had multiple tunnels and bunkers carved into its slopes of limestone for military purposes. An isolated ridge extending over 3 miles with six distinct peaks. Here, Kesselring and staff remained huddled until May 1944 when the Allies shoved them out.

Loyal, Kesselring was certainly a recipient of Hitler's largesse. It pleased the Führer to reward generals like Kesselring through sanctioned "enticements" (bribes), large sums of cash, cars, and estates emanating from Hitler's pocket, and he did this for many throughout the Third Reich. This was a generally accepted, outright practice of buying loyalty in Nazi Germany, and eyebrows remained unraised. No one but Hitler knew better how to maintain allegiance to *Führer und Vaterland:* "[Hitler] especially esteemed Bavarians from lower middle-class circumstances in contrast to the high officers of noble birth, especially linking highest technical efficiency of the former with cadaver-like obedience sinking into obsequiousness."

(The "incentives" did not always secure complete allegiance to Hitler, particularly for *Generalfeldmarschall* Erwin Rommel, who had been on the periphery of the failed attempt to assassinate the Führer on 20 July 1944. Rommel was coerced into suicide so his family could be allowed pension payments after his death. On 14 October 1944, the Desert Rat, as he was known, voluntarily bit into a cyanide capsule in the back seat of a plush staff car in a wooded area not far from his home in Herrlingen, a small village near Ulm in the state of Baden-Württemberg, Germany.)

For several weeks, Kesselring had been looking for a target like the harbor at Bari—something decisive, pivotal, that could provide a decisive blow to the Allies. He figured a definitive air strike on Bari would halt or delay the advance of the British Eighth Army and stall General Doolittle's newly formed Fifteenth Air Force. To himself and his staff, he knew he might be asking for the impossible—the Luftwaffe was lacking planes, pilots, supplies, and fuel; Kesselring kept this idea of bombing Bari to himself instead of wanting to hear ideas from his staff.

So, toward the end of November, he ordered a high-level conference at his headquarters. The food and wine were the best

Italy had, and the meeting room was "comfortably warm despite the cold Italian weather." The news from the front at this moment, however, was dreadful.

The British Eighth Army advanced almost ninety miles in the previous two weeks, attaining the Sangro River. The Fifth Army grabbed the entrance of the Liri Valley, which led to Rome. For now, the Americans had been stymied in front of the natural strongholds of Monte Camino, Monte Lungo, and Monte Sammucro—as soon as reinforcements arrived, the Allies and the Axis knew the battle would resume. Kesselring thought some way had to be found quickly to stop or slow down the British and the Americans. He was certain, too, that the collective minds at this gathering could devise a profitable plan for the Germans—and that it would be in align with his strategic notions.

Before the meeting convened, the attendees had informally agreed that there were three choices on the agenda for going on the offensive: bombing Doolittle's bombers of the new Fifteenth Air Force on the ground at Foggia, bombing the Fifth Army, or bombing Bari's harbor and ships and cutting off the supply lines to the Fifth and Eighth Armies.

Doolittle's Fifteenth Air Force was causing considerable trouble for the Germans. On 1 December, Fifteenth HQ had closed down in Tunis and moved to Bari (Foggia). Over 100 B-17s bombed the Turin ball-bearing works without losses or positive victories. That same day, B-26s with P-38 fighter escorts attacked bridges and railroad facilities at Auila, Cecina, and Sestri Levante. The next day, 2 December, in daylight, B-24s, with fighter escort, bombed the town area, marshaling yards and railroad bridges at Bolzano. B-26s achieved excellent results on the bridges of

Orvieto, and B-17s blasted submarine pens at Marseille. All of this, plus the potential the Fifteenth had for further hurting the Germans, was on everyone's mind when the meeting convened.

Attending the conference today, the revered *Generalfeldmsarshall* (General of the Army) Wolfram Karl Ludwig Moritz Hermann Freiherr von Richthofen, reporting directly to Kesselring and responsible for Luftwaffe air activity throughout Italy and Sicily. *Freiherr*, a rank of nobility that translates to "free lord" or "baron" in English, was a German World War I flying ace. "A competent but ruthless practitioner of air power" —a man who came from a long, honorable lineage of noblemen, including his distant cousin, the famous Red Baron, Manfred von Richthofen. (It was the Red Baron that inspired a pop song many years later, "Snoopy vs. the Red Baron," sung by The Royal Guardsmen and released in 1966. It was inspired by the Peanuts comic strip character Snoopy and his imaginary battles with the iconic Red Baron, a renowned World War I flying ace. In the comic strip, Snoopy often fantasizes about being a World War I flying ace himself, flying atop his doghouse in aerial combat against his arch-nemesis, the Red Baron.) Noted as a mercurial and independent general, the five-foot-six von Richthofen was ready to attempt any air strike at any time, as long as the odds were at least fifty-fifty in his favor.

In attendance, too, *Oberst* (Colonel) Werner Baumbach, general of the bombers. Tall, slender, blond, and seemingly out of a Hollywood casting office, the handsome *Oberst* had previously been given the task of completely reorganizing the German bomber fleet and turning the tides of the war. For this and his previous combat service, Hitler awarded him the Knight's Cross for the destruction of over 300,000 gross register tons of Allied shipping. As a fighter pilot, Baumbach had fought the RAF and the USAAF over the Continent and the Mediterranean as a pilot and a commander of a bomber *Gruppe* (Group). Now, Kesselring was asking him to perform a marvel—a big one.

Another astute officer attending the conference that Kesselring went to for vision and knowledge, Luftwaffe *Generalleutnant* (Major General) Dietrich Georg Magnus Peltz, a Hitler favorite, an expert on bombing—awarded the thirty-first Swords to his Knight's Cross on 23 July 1943 as *Oberst im Generalstab of Angriffsführer* (Colonel in the General Staff of Assault Leaders) England. Peltz brought his pioneering "Peltz Doctrine" to the meeting, a tactic he crafted and used successfully earlier in the war: Hitting a single target with a massive number of bombers rather than spreading thin the attack force. In 1939, Peltz was an *Oberleutenant* (First Lieutenant). Because of his excellent record, four years later, he rose to *Generalmajor* (Brigadier General), an unheard-of achievement in any army. He flew numerous combat missions over Greece, Russia, and Poland. Hitler personally "invited" him to join Kesselring's staff.

Sitting around the large oak table puffing on cigars and cigarettes, each officer and their staff presented ideas. It had not taken Baumbach long after his arrival at Mont Soratte to assess the situation and conclude that, unlike other cities in Italy, Bari had suffered little bombing damage, but because of its strategic position, it would play a pivotal role in supplying the Allies during the battle for Italy; von Richthofen and Kesselring agreed with this overall assessment.

Baumbach told the gathering that, up to today, Bari was doing well because the German's resources for bombing the harbor were running sparse—aircraft, aircrews, aviation, gas, bombs—that the Luftwaffe had to cherry-pick their targets and, till now, Bari was not one of those cherries. Little bomb damage, few casualties, and minimal disruption to daily living—all because of the Luftwaffe's inability to launch effective airstrikes, if any, against the harbor. Bari was a crucial Mediterranean hub supplying both the American Fifth and British Eighth Armies with vital supplies. Fact was that it supported almost a million Allied troops engaged in trying to drive the Germans out of Italy.

One of the grand buildings along the waterfront stood as the headquarters of the US Fifteenth Air Force, under the command of USAAF Brigadier General James H. "Jimmy" Doolittle, who led the audacious raid on Tokyo on 18 April 1942. Much to his resentment, Doolittle knew he was here in Bari only in a supporting, almost subservient, role; all his B-17s and B-24s were forty-five miles away at the Foggia airfields constantly hungering for fuel and parts coming through Bari's harbor. Their main mission was bombing targets north of Italy. Germany's communications, economic, and industrial sites were within striking distance of the Foggia airfields and were his main targets. "…44 percent of the enemy's [Germany's] crude and synthetic oil were less than 600 miles from Foggia."

Von Richthofen related one of the most important points of their conference: He told the participants that the Allies in Bari were over-confident, which he relished. Because confidence fosters hubris, and hubris minimizes significant details. He told the group that since the harbor was basically unscathed, the Americans and British, as well as the citizens of Bari, thought it was never going to be bombed; the Germans didn't have the resources or the willpower, they falsely imagined. Mostly, he asserted, they underestimated the German spirit.

Since the British controlled the harbor at Bari, they usually had the last word—often to the irritation of the Americans. This often led to ill-suited solutions and cracks in the armor. This head-butting and territorial imperative attitude led to many conflicts that did little to defend the harbor effectively.

Coincidentally, on the morning the Luftwaffe bombed Bari, 2 December 1943, British Air Marshal Sir Arthur "Mary" Coningham organized a press conference announcing that Bari was all but "immune from attack" from the Luftwaffe. Coningham's precipitous announcement could not have been more inauspicious and would leave a double dollop of egg on the air marshal's handsome face. (Interestingly, there are several theories why Coningham had the nickname "Mary": the most common was that Mary is a play on "Māori" due to his New Zealand background.) At the press conference, Coningham rashly announced to the assembled reporters—to the world—that the Royal Air Force had "knocked out" the Axis forces in the Mediterranean, adding emphatically: "I would regard it as a personal affront and insult if the Luftwaffe should attempt any significant action in the area." Hours later that night, 109 Ju 88s dropped over 105 tons of bombs on the port city. This was a dreadful blunder on Coningham's part that caused many guffaws in Kesselring's high command, particularly those on his immediate staff. Coningham would only have to wait a scant few hours to personally witness a catastrophic attack of the first level—similar to the Japanese attack on Pearl Harbor two years previously (almost to the day).

From this date forward Air Marshal Coningham would be dealing with severe political headwinds for the remainder of his career. At the end of June 1944, Field Marshal Bernard Montgomery asked soon-to-be-promoted general of the Army General Dwight D. Eisenhower at Supreme Allied Headquarters for Coningham's removal after Coningham criticized the army for tardiness in capturing Caen to make available airfields for tactical aircraft; this was denied.

As he recited his opening statement and took reporters' questions, his words were underlined by Bari's harbor bristling and throbbing with unprecedented activity that would come to a sudden, disastrous halt at 7:30 that evening.

Accounts differ, but there were approximately thirty Allied ships—Polish, British, Dutch, American, Norwegian, and others—crammed into the harbor, taking up every useable water surface within the ancient breakwaters and antiquated docks. The ships had to be guided to their moorings by harbor pilots and then nestled against each other's gunwales, or the seawalls and piers, sardines in a can—this was a mistake forced by the circumstances of the harbor and should have been disallowed by the US Navy that would bear partial responsibility later for the disaster. The explosion of one ship had the potential to seriously damage adjacent ships and so on or set them ablaze—which would happen. The dock hands had been humping 24/7, and the usual blackout on the night of 2 December would be suspended. The lights left aglow all night long—a sparkling beacon, an unintended navigational aid for the German bombers, which delighted the pilots.

This massive infusion of supplies the ships were offloading would be applied to the Allies' pending efforts to begin a push north in January 1944—a massive effort to press the Germans beyond Rome and eventually out of Italy. Both the Allies and Kesselring knew what the speed bump was: the so-called Gustav Line. This Allied effort to get there and beyond would require enormous amounts of military equipment and matériel: ammunition, aviation fuel, medical supplies, food, tanks, armored personnel carriers, and ambulances topped off with fuel and ready to roll. All this accumulated in and around the picturesque Bari harbor. On the quayside berths, numerous mountains of supplies were growing to storied heights. Boxes of ammunition, artillery shells, and medical supplies rose high on the stone moles (a quay or a jetty, not a furry animal), a sign of the heavy fighting that was anticipated. The Americans had led a six-month-long campaign that did not merge—it had been raging since 10 July 1943. What was planned had to be successful and final, and these supplies coming into the harbor were crucial.

Kesselring, showing his famous skeletal smile and impecunious teeth, says to Peltz, "If we can take out Bari, we stand an excellent chance of recapturing the entire Foggia airfield complex and negating the effectiveness of Doolittle's bombers."

"The Fifteenth will be deprived of essential supplies," a staff member says.

"This is a propitious moment," adds Baumbach.

Then Richthofen presents a realistic but problematic note: "The only large number of planes I have left for such an attack are my Ju 88s based in the north. Perhaps I could put 150 in the air immediately."

Peltz, without hesitation, admits that the notion of attacking

Bari has serious merit; he's enthused. He says, "Anything that can be done to delay or destroy the Fifteenth Air Force would be pivotal and advantageous to Germany." However, the paramount question continued: Is it possible under current circumstances to launch an air strike that would result in slowing down the Allies on the ground and in the air?

For the next sixty minutes, the four officers discuss the feasibility and problems of bombing Bari. Aides scurry back and forth, gathering and collating reports from embedded spies who have continually observed the numbers of ships, types of cargo they were offloading, and the time it takes to turn ships around after their loads are put ashore.

Then, a wonderful revelation.

A staff officer enters the room and hands a piece of paper to von Richthofen.

"*Herren*," von Richthofen announces, after reading the brief typewritten note and grinning, "the antiaircraft aiming device that Bari has on the roof of the Margherita Theater is undergoing repairs; it is out of action." This device was attached to Swedish-designed Bofors 40mm guns around Bari, more commonly referred to as ack-ack guns, and was the only such aiming device in Bari.

Toward the meeting's end, Kesselring goes around the table—and wants opinions from each of the generals enjoying his wine and cigars.

After a few minutes, he gets a consensus: not only destroy all the ships anchored in the harbor but hit them so hard that some of the ships sink, causing obstructions to other ships trying to navigate the harbor—and thus disallow ships from leaving for replenishment elsewhere.

The lack of firepower on the ground adds to Bari's vulnerability. Further, the Royal Air Force fighters stationed at Foggia are also unavailable to help Bari.

Now, Bari has almost nothing formidable to defend itself—an egregious oversight of the first order: no antiaircraft guns, no fighters—except for near-impotent long rifles, shotguns, and handguns of the police and citizenry, and deck guns on some of the Liberty Ships. Further, Naval Armed Guard contingents aboard American Liberty Ships in the harbor had been ordered *not* to fire at enemy aircraft. A British officer ordered a US Navy ensign: "In case of enemy air attack, he was to coordinate his fire with a radar-controlled shore gun firing white tracers." What prompted the order was a concern for lack of coordination among the ships in port and several reasons given by the ship's commanders: fear of exploding ships loaded with ammunition and other volatile supplies would make the use of defensive weaponry risky. Further, the commanders feared that firing antiaircraft weapons could trigger explosions if munitions in the ships were hit, either by enemy fire or by falling wreckage from destroyed aircraft. Also, strict secrecy and security measures were a concern: at the time of the attack, Bari was packed with twenty-seven Liberty ships carrying classified cargo. Among these—containing the most sensitive secret of all—was the SS *John Harvey*, an American Liberty ship, which carried a clandestine cargo unknown to almost everyone—especially the Germans with their spies and extensive intelligence apparatus in and around the harbor.

And that's why von Richthofen wanted Renz and his Me

210 over Bari on a spying mission every day for five consecutive days: to check the day-by-day, almost minute-by-minute progress of the Allied activities in and around Bari's harbor—to note how it expanded and contracted over five days. Renz's arrival times over Bari would vary, presenting a slice of each day's activities, cargos, and progress.

Von Richthofen and Kesselering had a mutually clear picture of how important Bari's harbor was as soon as Renz returned from his last recon over the harbor.

Kesselring leans forward, balances his fat cigar on an ashtray, orders von Richthofen to prepare every bomber he has in northern Italy, and craft an immediate plan to bomb Bari's harbor.

Von Richthofen says, "I *have* a plan already crafted, *Heer Generalfeldmarschall*."

"I'm sure you do, Wolfram."

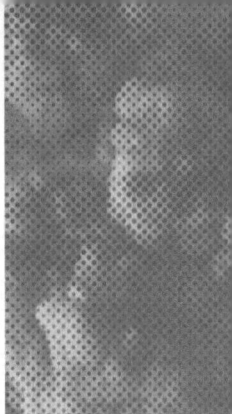

2

LIBERTY SHIPS

Driving southeast from Grosseto Airport to Bari takes nearly six hours.

Flying at 250 mph in his Me 210 will take *Hauptmann* Renz about an hour and a half, and then he'll be over the Bari harbor for the last time. There, he will fly a racetrack pattern over the ships mostly, taking pictures and making notes.

At the Grosseto airfield, Renz signals Hurdelbrink, and the sergeant jerks away the wooden chocks from the tires.

In the Me 210 cockpit, Renz clicks the ignition switch to the Start position for the Daimler-Benz number one engine, the one that needed an oil top-off. The propeller spins once, twice, herky-jerky, and pillows of blue smoke curl away from the exhaust stacks, and the air crackles and explodes. Stutters again. In a few seconds, the RPMs smooth out and the engine is running. Renz eyeing it suspiciously. He repeats the procedure for the second engine.

He monitors engine gauges for proper oil pressure, engine RPMs, and temperature.

Adjusts the throttle slightly to increase RPMs to a stable idle setting.

Repeats for the second engine.

So far, so good, he thinks. The Hag has not fallen apart in place.

He sits staring at the gauges allowing the engines to warm up at low RPM; the oil temperature and pressure stabilize across all engine systems. A typical warm-up period is from 3 to 5 minutes. This warm-up is crucial to ensure that the engine oil reaches the proper temperature and viscosity, reducing wear and tear on the engine components. Apparently, the Hag doesn't pay attention to Veit's impatience. The process allows time for him to double-check that all engine functions are performing correctly before takeoff.

Renz thought that perhaps he would get a commendation for his five reconnaissance flights over Bari, not the Knight's Cross or anything lofty like that—maybe a sterling silver Honor Goblet of the Luftwaffe (*Ehrenpokal der Luftwaffe*), also referred to as an Honor Goblet For Special Achievement in the Air War, engraved with the recipient's name, rank and date. It would look good on his mantel after the war.

The Me 210 bobs and bumps for the runway, and Renz peeks at the panel clock.

Renz's rear gunner, *Oberfeldwebel* (Master Sergeant) Dieter Jürgens, has been handpicked for this mission. Aside from being a superb gunner, Jürgens operates the aircraft's defensive armaments, has a superb situational eye, is a good communicator, and an expert on the Hag's intricate systems.

Jürgens will be the prime camera operator shooting as many pictures as possible—if they get back to Grosett or the Hag kills them first.

Veit Renz can fly down to Bari with his eyes closed today, as he has done four times over the past four days. Gives the Hag the juice and taxis out to the runway.

And off they go, unknowingly lofting into a historic mission that will be little noted in history books. Veit sets up a rate of ascent for approximately 500 to 600 feet per minute. This is relatively modest compared to more successful fighters of the era, who could often climb at rates exceeding 1,000 feet per minute. But the Me 210's performance was affected by its heavy armament and armor, which were designed to support its roles as a heavy fighter and attack aircraft. Veit avoids flying over land as much as he can, flying mostly over the Adriatic.

When he reaches altitude, Veit is amazed—the Hag's engines haven't exploded, she has not demanded a Dutch roll, the sound of her exhaust is smooth as honeybees, and the notorious troublesome aircraft not doing anything erratic or dubious. He reaches for his coffee, takes a gulp. Then a bite of Weisswurst. He says to his number One engine, "*Don't look at me that way. I'm trusting you so far.*" And the engine winks back.

Renz can see in his mind *Generalfeldmarsahll* Richtofen standing by, twiddling his thumbs, waiting for the final report. Right now, all available Luftwaffe Ju 88s are gassed up, loaded with bombs at the scattered airports in northern Italy, the crews sitting around the dispersal areas smoking, snoozing—ready to take off. Set a course to Bari.

He checks the panel clock again. The oil discrepancy has put him behind schedule. He sets up a steep descent north of the Manfredonia spur. Rolls the trim tab forward and starts a gradual descent, picking up airspeed, working the trim tabs as the Hag slices through the air.

Then, here comes the coastline west of Foggia.

A big mistake that nearly gets them killed.

Two bright flashes of light catch his eye, and he thinks it's his imagination and blinks his eyes, clearing them.

But it is not your imagination, Hauptmann *Renz.*

He looks again, and the bright flashes are black dots flying in a classic wingman formation.

His pilot's mind, his intuition, his experience tell him exactly what they are.

"*Kämpfer!*"

Fighters!

Twin engines, twin-vertical stabilizers.

Glinting like sterling silver knives in the sun.

They had not been painted olive drab yet, so they must have just arrived in Italy.

New and efficient.

Two USAAF P-38 Lightnings came at him with an M2 .20mm canon mounted in the nose and four .50 caliber machine guns—a formidable array of weaponry that can easily rip apart a Me 210.

Renz has erased the notion of the Honor Goblet.

Slams the throttles forward. Feels the punch of acceleration.

Gets maximum manifold pressure and RPM. Praying the Hag's engines will behave.

Then, noses over, does a split S, and heads for the water, barely skimming the shimmering surface. He's in evasive mode now, climbing, diving, S turning. The P-38s don't let up, *oh, no, brother, we're coming for you!*

Outside his cockpit window, bullets smack and spray the water. Renz jukes and canters the Me 210. Then, *deus ex machina,* "God from the machine" east of Jasto—the P-38s give up the chase, just like that, gray exhaust plumes marking their pernicious flight as they peel up and scream away and away and away.

Probably low on fuel, Renz thinks, *and my flying skills.*

Waiting for Renz is Bari's harbor.

At 10,000 feet, he dips the left wing for an unobstructed view. He's a few miles away from the harbor and is slightly off course. He lowers the nose and rolls back the elevator trim. When he comes level he can clearly make out the distinctive outline of the harbor. It appears like a ragged O with the entrance at the eleven o'clock position. And just a bit east, the "Bambino" Stadium—nicknamed as a reward to the citizens of Bari for having the most male births in Italy. All around the city, the war-weary citizenry strolling, dining anticipating the coming Christmas holiday. But it is the harbor that grabs Renz's focus.

He flies northeast, then sets up the racetrack pattern over the harbor and city at 10,000 feet. He's quick and deft with the controls, and the Hag doesn't seem to mind that a master is flying her. Like yesterday, the *Oberleutenant* will make three passes—one north to south, the other east to west. Then zooms back home with his final report. He presses his intercom button to notify Jürgens what the process will be today—the same as yesterday. The same sky. The same harbor. The same butterflies in his stomach. The same. The same. The same.

Renze flies straight and steady into the top of the imaginary pattern, the West Jetty. The jetty, or mole, is part of the harbor's mouth, with open water separating it from the East Jetty. Here, the Adriatic and the harbor merge, forming an entrance. Renz points south maintaining 10,000 feet, going toward Molo Pizzoli and Molo San Vito jetties. Here, scattered in a disciplined manner, Renz and Dieter Jürgens, the machine gunner sitting behind Renz, begin taking pictures and making notes. While noting as much as they can, Renz has the Hag flying a straight line south toward the Stazione Marittima, which houses the Allied War Shipping Administration Office; they note this, both of them simultaneously.

Most of the merchant ships are anchored, bow in, at the East Jetty and no more than two feet apart from each other. They are US Liberty ships referred to among seamen as "draught horses" because they convey characteristics of strength, endurance, and reliability attributed to big work horses with hairy hoofs; they are also referred to as Ugly Ducklings, or, as President Roosevelt described them, "Dreadful Looking Objects." The patrician Roosevelt more aligned with the graceful, expensive lines of haughty yachts that his membership at the American Yacht Club in Rye, New York, affords him. In 1936, Congress passed the Merchant Marine Act, which became the cornerstone of its shipbuilding program. America needed merchant marine capability, particularly in wartime, and the capacity to carry troops and war materials. Before WWII started, the Act required five-hundred ships to be built over ten years. The US Maritime Commission saw to it that this building venture was met.

Within a year and a half after the United States entered the war in 1941, the twelve major shipyards in the United States were building ships faster than the enemy could sink them. From 1942 through 1945, United States shipyards built 5,592 merchant ships, of which 2,701 were Liberty ships, 414 were the fast Victory type, 651 were tankers, 417 were standard cargo ships, and the remaining 1,400 were military or minor types.

Such was the need so urgent that one Liberty Ship, the S.S. *Robert E. Peary*, was built *and* launched in an astonishing four and a half days.

The mission was quite simple—get the material delivered.

In fact, they were built in large numbers to be expendable—the more built, the more they got through with their cargo. "If a ship got through and was then sunk, it was declared a success and worthwhile." When merchant seamen heard this, their happiness did not flourish.

Typically, crews on a Liberty Ship consisted of approximately forty merchant mariners: captain (master); the deck department consisting of the chief officer, deck cadet, first, second, and third officers, boatswain, carpenter, able bodies and ordinary seamen; radio operator; steward's department consisting of a chief steward, cooks, galley and messmen; purser; and the engine room, department: chief engineer, engine room cadet, first, second and third engineers, water tender, firemen, oilers, and wipers.

On almost every cruise, merchant ships had to face a variety of threats from armed Raiders, kamikaze-like attacks, mines, and submarines. The facts presented the grim reality of these forays:

12,000 men were wounded, at least 1100 died from their wounds, and more than 600 men and women were taken prisoner. In prison camps or aboard Japanese ships while being transported to other camps, 70 died through a variety of gruesome ways. Some were incinerated, some froze to death, some starved and drowned. More than 31 ships simply disappeared. For those thinking sailing the seas on merchant ships was easy duty, remember this: one in 26 mariners serving aboard these ships in the second world war suffered a larger percentage of war-related deaths than all other US services. This information was kept top secret from the enemy to hide their success. The secret was also kept from potential draftees.

Almost every week, the newspapers carried just about the same distracting, inaccurate story: two medium sized allied ships sunk in the Atlantic." Realistically, in 1942 the average was over 30 ships per week.

Each ship (not all the ships were Liberty Ships) was protected by approximately twenty-eight men of the United States Naval armed Guard. The Naval Armed Guard and the Merchant Marine, present in Bari's harbor on the night of 2 December, suffered terrible casualties during and after the bombing.

* * *

Hauptmann Renz has configured the Hag to hold the top of a racetrack pattern above the East Jetty at 10,000 feet and 230 mph, trimming the ailerons and elevator to hold steady at that altitude. At that moment, in front of the Hotel Albergo Oriente, two eyewitnesses glance up and see the Me 210's contrail. Unaccustomed to bombing attacks and reconnaissance missions, the eyewitnesses have no idea what the aircraft is doing; they are civilians. They are part of the general lethargy of the ancient city that doesn't seem to mind too much that WWII is flaming all around them.

One of them says, "Don't worry, there are never bombing attacks on Bari."

Renz and Jürgen now have an excellent bird's eye view of the harbor and the ships; they take pictures and continue making notes and drawings and memorizing the ships' positions.

Although this is not a complete listing of the ships moored in the harbor, here are some of the most notable vessels—not all were US Liberty Ships. One, the USS *Aroostok*, was a US naval cargo ship.

The SS *Joseph Wheeler* is moored at berth 28 at the East Jetty, fully burdened with ammunition in a variety of calibers. The ship had the distinction of being named for the only Confederate States of America soldier to be appointed to the rank of general who fought at Bunker Hill in the Spanish-American War. General Wheeler served in the US House of Representatives from Alabama's 8th District and was a graduate of the United States Military Academy. The *Wheeler* had been torpedoed months before docking at Bari in December and was deliberately run aground to salvage its cargo. Months later, the *Wheeler* sailed for Bari from New York on 11 November 1943 in Convoy UGS023, arriving in Bari on 1 December via Augusta, Sicily, and Taranto, Italy.

The USS *Aroostock* (AOG-14), an American naval ship, and the third to take the name of a river in Northern Maine. Launched in December 1937, she was a tanker for the Esso Corporation and then became a US Navy ship in April 1943. When she sailed into the Bari harbor aboard was a formidable cargo: 19,000 barrels of highly volatile 100-octane gasoline. Most notable and duly crucial because it was destined solely for General Doolittle's Fifteenth Air Force thirsting bombers. The gasoline would be unloaded at Bari and then pumped through pipelines to the Foggia Airfields. The captain of the *Aroostock*, W. R. Hayes, was anxious because he could not unload his hazardous cargo. Anchored 300 to 350 yards off the Cataldo mole, the *Aroostook* wallows in the heavily congested area of merchant ships.

The Liberty Ship SS *John Bascom* was named after a person of distinction: college president, sociologist, philosopher, and nineteenth-century educator. The cargo consisted of 8,300 tons of foodstuffs, acid, high-test gasoline in 50-gallon drums, and Army hospital equipment. Going toward Bari on 1 November 1943, the ship neared Gibraltar, hounded by submarines and German planes dropping depth charges ahead of the convoy. When the ship sailed up the boot of Italy on the Adriatic, those aboard had no idea of their destination—it was top secret. But as they neared the port of Bari, Cadet Midshipmen Leroy C. Heinse "heard antiaircraft guns and a reconnaissance plane flying over the port seeking targets. That was the tip-off, so to speak, that something was going to happen…"

The SS *Samuel J. Tilden* sailed from New York on 14 July 1943 in Convoy UGS 15 and anchored in Gibraltar for twenty days. The Liberty Ship was named after a 19th-century politician, governor, publisher, and unsuccessful presidential candidate. The ship's cargo consisted of trucks with full gasoline tanks in No. 4 and No. 5 holds. On deck, 6,000 gallons of high octane gasoline were stored in the No. 2 hold, 100 tons of ammunition stored in No. 4 and No. 5 holds, a deck cargo of gasoline in drums, and five hospital units, also on board were 209 military passengers; 186 US Army personnel and 23 British Army personnel. One of the Naval Armed Guards remembered that the *Tilden* "had a deck load of mustard gas. This gas was in metal containers and very plainly printed, MUSTARD GAS, on the sides of the containers." This was not the only Liberty Ship that brought mustard gas into Bari's harbor. It would be the last.

The Liberty Ship *John Harvey* would always be known as the epicenter of the tragedy at Bari on 2 December 1943.

Notable at birth, notable at death.

The *Harvey* was distinguished from the beginning of her short, historic life: she was named after one of the signers of the Articles of Confederation. In 1777, John Harvey was also a member of the Continental Congress. The ship sailed from Baltimore on her fourth and final trip. There, she loaded a secret cargo of mustard gas. Two thousand M47A1-100 lb. bombs were loaded secretly from the Easter Chemical Warfare Depot to Curtis Bay Depot and finally to the Baltimore Cargo Port. So secret and so sensitive, the *Harvey* had her own safety crew of seven men to ensure proper handling and secrecy. In charge was a cargo security officer, Lieutenant Thomas H. Richardson.

So secret was the cargo that the master of the *John Harvey*, Elwin F. Knowles, was not told (officially) that his ship was loaded with mustard gas. But Captain Knowles, a seasoned skipper, knew better. After loading the lethal shipment, the *Harvey* sailed for Norfolk on 15 October and arrived in Orang on 2 November in Convoy UGS 21.

Copies of *Harvey's* manifest were signed by the Docks Superintendent at Bari on 25 November. No record of them has been found; there is no trace and no evidence that they were distributed to the proper authorities. It is almost certain that they were deliberately destroyed.

According to a *British Most Secret Report:*

On the 26th [sic, should be 28] or 29 November a representative of the US Port Office went on board the John Harvey and was told by the Security Officer [not Knowles] that he had a cargo of mustard gas.

There is some evidence that the presence of a cargo of mustard was discussed between the Docks Superintendent, the Acting Port Commandant, and the Sea Transport Officer, and it was considered in view of her [the John Harvey] low priority and the berthing space available, that she was in as safe as a place as she could be found.

Neither NOIC nor Comd. No. 6 Base Sub area was aware before the raid that the John Harvey contained toxic ammunition.

Apparently, the mustard gas cargo was so sacrosanct that no group, no entity except the Safety Crew, knew that a massive amount of mustard gas packed aboard the *John Harvey*. This secret would linger "officially" long after WWII ended. Meanwhile, because it was unknown, ineffective medical treatments were administered, and many people died unnecessarily after the bombing. Nevertheless, because it was secret and Knowles was supposed to be unaware of its presence, he was unable to get the ship in position to offload its cargo ASAP.

Each day that Renz flew over the harbor—this would be his fifth and last mission—he was amazed at what he saw down on the water: thirty-seven ships today, including ships from the United Kingdon, Poland, the United States, Norway, and the Netherlands. Some days, there would be fewer, others more, and the numbers from various countries would vary. He is surprised by two things: Bari's complacency and the volume of supplies shipping into the harbor every day. It seems difficult to imagine how the Germans will win this war. In the back of his mind, he is astounded by the vast materiel the Allies could produce: the supplies on those ships were intended to defeat his country, Germany, and he cannot see the limit to what the Allies have and what they could ship. Renz is a practical person: he knows the Luftwaffe will probably destroy every ship in the harbor, probably tonight, and cause a massive amount of damage and death and slow down the Allies' efforts. At the same time, he knows it would only be a matter of time before the Allies were back with more ships and more supplies. This bombing would not be a so-called magic bullet, not the bombing some expected to end the war. In his fighter pilot's mind, the raid tonight will only postpone the inevitable. First and foremost, however, he is a soldier of the Reich who had taken an oath to serve his country and that he will do.

Now, the Me 210 comes hard around the top of the racetrack pattern just over the West Jetty.

To Veit Renz and Dieter Jurgens, it is quite evident that the amount of ships in the harbor today has increased since yesterday—since the first day of their reconnaissance. While they cannot discern the names of the ships, they both count and diagram 27 (approximately) ships from a variety of countries. This is guess work on their part because Renz has to fly the Hag and scribble with his pencil. Still, when their report is given, their estimation and nationalities of the ships will sync with the spies the Germans have around the city and the harbor.

After spending ten minutes over the harbor, flying the racetrack pattern twice, taking pictures, and drawing, Renz sets a course northeast to their base and orders Jurgens to send a coded message via Morse code. Essentially, there are four more ships in the packed harbor today. Most notable. Further, Renz writes on his knee pad: *Keine Kampfflugzeuge*. No fighter aircraft. That is another significant point for the attack tonight.

Renz thinks that if the Allies, the force down in Bari were diligent, they would have designed defenses around the city. Instead, the calm they are experiencing is an indication of the tiredness that will harm them with a severity they have not imagined.

A few seconds later, the code reaches von Richthofen, who notifies Kesselring, who orders his Ju 88 crews to prepare to bomb Bari. Kesselring is delighted. His tooth grin betrays his disposition.

Then Kesselring signals, and the bombing of Bari harbor commences.

This mission will be the start of a kerfuffle the world had never before seen, and not even the morose Anaxagoras, the ancient Greek philosopher, if bonused all the time in the universe, will not sort out for some time.

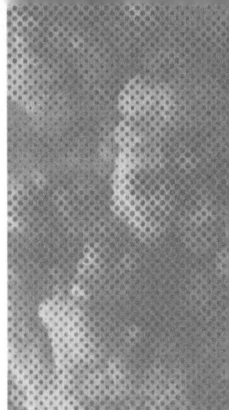

3

HENRY CRONBACH LOWENHAUPT

The Italian Campaign of World War II began on July 10, 1943, when Allied forces, consisting mainly of American and British troops, launched an invasion of Sicily in an operation known as Operation Husky. This initial invasion aimed to remove the Axis powers from the island, which they accomplished by mid-August 1943.

Following the success in Sicily, the Allies continued their push into mainland Italy. They landed on the Italian peninsula on September 3, 1943, and Italy officially surrendered on September 8, 1943. However, German forces continued to resist in Italy, leading to a prolonged and difficult start and end of the Italian campaign.

The Italian Campaign was notable for its harsh conditions and the tough, mountainous terrain, which made the fighting particularly grueling for both sides, Allies and Germans.

The exact numbers of troops stationed in Italy during the Italian Campaign fluctuated significantly due to various phases of the Campaign, reinforcements, and casualties. However, at the peak of the Campaign, the United States had multiple divisions engaged. Initially, during the landing in Sicily and later on the Italian mainland, there were around 250,000 American troops involved. As the campaign progressed, this number varied, with additional troops being deployed or shifted to other fronts, like the upcoming invasion of Normandy in June 1944.

Contrary to popular believe, not every G.I. in Italy (or any battlefield) during this period carried a gun and was engaged in combat.

In Italy at this time, as in other countries, the distribution of combat versus support roles varied, but a common rule of thumb for the U.S. Army was approximately ten percent of personnel were in direct combat roles, while the remaining ninety percent were in support roles. This ratio, often referred to as the "tooth-to-tail" ratio, is a military term that refers to the amount of military personnel it takes to support combat troops (the "tail") compared to the number of combat troops themselves (the "tooth"). A higher ratio indicates a larger support or logistical element compared to the number of troops directly involved in combat roles. This ratio is used to assess the efficiency of military logistics and operations, indicating how well resources are being utilized to support combat effectiveness.It also highlights the significant portion of military personnel dedicated to logistics, administration, medical care, communications, and other support functions essential for the operations of those in combat roles.

Among the American troops in Italy between January 1943 and 1945 was Henry Cronbach Lowenhaupt, born in St. Louis, Missouri on April 3, 1913. His parents were Abraham Lowenhaupt and Bessie Cronbach Lowenhaupt. Henry graduated from Soldan High School in St. Louis and was admitted to Harvard College in 1933 when he was sixteen years, a formidable achievement. After graduating, he walked across the street and entered Harvard Law School, graduating in 1936. He then joined the law firm founded by his father, Abraham, the first lawyer in the United States to concentrate in federal tax law.

While in high school, Henry belonged to the Writer's Club and the Mathematics Club. His letters home from Italy during the war show his inclination unusual skill, for superb writing. During 1943 and 1945, Henry wrote hundreds of letters with a prodigious output of nearly 108,000 words.

In a taped Interview on February 6, 1986, Henry, explains his exceptional journey to from Harvard College to Harvard Law School. This interview was put into a Lowenhaupt family book:

> "One day after school," Henry said in the taped interview, "the principal called us into his office—this was in our senior year. He asked each of us, 'All those interested in going to college, raise your hands.' And then asked each of us where wanted to go to college. He'd say, 'That's a good choice. I'll get you in there.' If he thought someone was not qualified, he'd tell them something like, 'We'll talk about that later,' or maybe, 'We can find something better for you.' But when he came to me, I

told him I wanted to go to Harvard. Because then, like today, Harvard was well known as one of the most prestigious colleges in the country. I had absolutely no reason for saying Harvard except I knew of its reputation—I just blurted it out. So, I was surprised when he said, 'Henry, Harvard is a good choice for you. I'll get you in. Don't bother taking the examinations.' We applied, and in due time, I got a letter saying I was admitted to Harvard College—can you imagine that happening today? I think that was a much better system than we have now."

During his time in the Army, Henry wrote a lot.

"The Constitutional History of England always intrigued me," he said, and "I took a lot of that."

At this time, Henry was thinking about a teaching career. But after all was said and done, like his lawyer father, he thought seriously about practicing law and working in his father's law firm in St. Louis.

Again, from the taped interview, Henry says, "That was easily accomplished in those days. The policy then was easy—they admitted almost everybody who asked and flunked about a third of them out after the first year."

When Henry entered Harvard in 1933, Franklin Delano Roosevelt was inaugurated as the 32nd president.

Prohibition came to an end with Utah, as the necessary 36th state, ratified on December 5 the 21st Amendment that repealed the 18th Amendment.

Lynchings again engaged the public's attention.

Maryland Governor Richie shocked many when he condoned a lynching in San Jose. In Missouri, a Black man was the victim of lynching in spite of the presence of troops.

Radio City Music Hall, a towering 70-floor office building in Rockefeller Center in New York, opened with an exhibition showing the first thirteen years of radio progress.

In baseball, the All-Star game was originated in Chicago.

Adolf Hitler came to power in Germany as Chancellor of the Third Reich. The next year, he became *Der Führer*. When this occurred, Henry and much of the rest of the world came to realize that war was almost inevitable.

People were lining up to see the year's big movies: *King Kong,* starring a very large gorilla named Kong; *Gold Diggers of 1933,* with Dick Powell and Ruby Keeler; and *Tugboat Annie,* with Marie Dressler and Wallace Beery.

And if you were listening to the radio, you probably learned the lyrics to *Let's Fall in Love, Stormy Weather,* and *Smoke Gets in Your Eyes.*

Three years later, in 1936, Henry graduated from Harvard Law School and went to work at his father's law firm in St. Louis, Missouri—at that time called Lowenhaupt and Waite. Henry went on to become a highly esteemed thirty-year practicing lawyer.

Everyone throughout the world, in 1933, sensed that a war was inevitable, with Hitler doing much to stir a pot of conflict and aggression.

At this time, the U.S. Army started to expand its ranks.

Henry said in the interview, "I was starting to wonder whether or not I could tolerate being in the Army. I mean, it was inevitable that, sooner or later, I was going to be drafted. So, I thought it might be better if I volunteered for something rather than sitting around for the axe to fall. But I sat around waiting too long. In due time, I got a notice. The United States Army wanted me."

After Henry arrived at the induction center, the doctor asked him, "How are you doing, Mr. Lowenhaupt?"

Henry said, "Very well, thank you, doctor."

"That's all I want to know."

Next, the Army took the recruit's clothes and, naked, piled them into a truck and drove twenty miles to Leavenworth, Kansas.

"This was a silly experience. There I was, a Harvard graduate, riding naked in an Army truck," Henry said in his 1986 taped interview.

Henry finally wound up at Jefferson Barracks and was issued a set of Army uniforms.

"This was basic training for college grads like me. I gave them my civilian clothes, and they gave me a set of Army uniforms—at least I didn't have to go naked anymore. The whole thing was a silly experience."

Henry learned to type at Jefferson Barracks. He figured, rightfully so, that having a typing skill in the U.S. Army was a rare skill—"I was something scarce in the Army," he said. "I was filing and typing and learned to become sufficiently efficient, and after a while, I could leave every day around three o'clock until the next day." Provided the time gone was less than 24 hours, Henry could sign his pass.

So, did he work in the morning when he came back?

"Of course not, I just loafed around. In fact, I got so bored I applied for OCS, Officer Candidate School, and was sent to adjutant general school in Washington, D.C. When I finished that, I didn't learn anything and got extremely bored just sitting around. One day, I was sitting around, and a friend of mine asked me if I wanted to go abroad. Guy's name was Bill Clark. "OCS was a strange place. One day, I got called to a so-called 'secret' meeting. They wanted to know if a boy in the bunk next to mine, Henry Levy, was a Communist. He was no more a Communist than I was. Back then, they were doing that kind of stuff—snooping around your background trying to weed out Communists. I knew that Levy was pretty much dissatisfied with the Army, but who wasn't? Everybody called the barracks 'The Land of Hell's Half Acre.' I think I was too old for it, but I never had any problems. At any rate, when they said who wanted to go overseas, I was bored stiff. I looked to Bill Clark, and he looked bored stiff, too, and I said let's volunteer, and we raised our hands. So off we went. We spent about a month on the way. Had no idea what our destination was."

But for the sailors on the ship, Henry was alone.

"Except for a rather stupid sergeant who was always telling me how he wasn't going to stay in the Army and that he was going to be sent back home immediately."

After many days at sea, Henry learned that he was aboard the ship carrying the bomb that was going to be used to blow up an important dam on the Rhine River. The one in a cargo hold of Henry's ship was among several "blockbusters" officially known as "HC" (High Capacity) bombs. Although Henry did not know it, and if he did, he could not write about it, these blockbuster bombs were part of an intricate plan to destroy German infrastructure, including potentially the dams along the Rhine River. This plan involved the use of the "bouncing bomb," developed by British engineer Barnes Wallis. The bombs were designed to bounce over water, evading torpedo nets before sinking against a dam wall and exploding. The most famous operation using these bouncing bombs was "Operation Chastise," carried out by the Royal Air Force's 617 Squadron, known as the Dam Busters. Turned into a film in 1955, it starred Richard Todd as Wing Commander Guy Gibson and Michael Redgrave as Barnes Wallis, the inventor of the "bouncing bomb" shaped like a massive 50-gallon oil drum. On the night of May 16-17, 1943, the 617 Squadron attacked dams in the Ruhr Valley, including the Möhne, Eder, and Sorpe dams. The Möhne and Eder dams were successfully breached, causing significant flooding and damage to German industrial capacity. While the primary targets were the Ruhr Valley dams, the concept and technology were rightfully considered for other strategic uses, including potential use against other infrastructure targets like bridges or additional dams along the Rhine River. They were designed to cause maximum damage over large areas, particularly against enemy cities and industrial targets. Named "blockbuster" because of its ability to destroy an entire city block in one hit. They ranged in size from 1,000 pounds to over 12,000 pounds, with the larger sizes introduced as the war progressed.

 Henry had no idea that he was aboard a ship carrying top-secret bombs and simultaneously sailing into WWII history books.

 While Henry was aboard in the Mediterranean, he saw a ship sink and describes it in a letter, "about one hundred yards from us—a very impressive sight to see a ship blow up and sink into the water backward." The ship was loaded with French Foreign Legion soldiers who were picturesque and completely panic-stricken. They should have dropped off the ship, as any fool could plainly see, but they stayed on and hung on to anything they could until the back rail broke and they slid off. "They went down after the ship, so I think there were ten or twelve out of a thousand that survived. It didn't scare me. It impressed me."

While on the ship, everyone had a job, a battle station. Henry was assigned to an anti-aircraft gun aboard the ship and was trying to figure out how to use the gun to shoot a submarine if necessary. "I couldn't figure out how to deflect the barrel to shoot a sub which was lower than the gunwales on our ship. A fellow came up to me and said, 'First, you're going to need your helmet. You might catch a cold.' So I put my helmet on. That's what I remember mostly about the trip."

After a long cruise around England and through the Mediterranean, Henry felt land under his feet at Algiers, the capital of Algeria, nicknamed "Algiers the White" because the buildings, seen from the sea, glistened silvery and lustrous. There, Henry checked in to the Hotel St. George, the Allied Forces Headquarters. General Eisenhower set up his headquarters there after the successful Operation Torch, which was the Allied invasion of North Africa. For a while, Henry lived at the hotel comfortably as a second lieutenant in the US Army.

"The St. George," Henry said, "was a luxurious old hotel situated in a big, splendid park. Eisenhower was there with his 'driver and secretary,' Kay Summersby, whom everyone seemed to know was his girlfriend. During World War II, there were rumors and speculations about the nature of their relationship, but I don't think it was confirmed that they were romantically involved. From here, I moved from this luxurious living to the headquarters of TUCOR [Theater Unspecified Category of Replacements or Theater Unit Construction, or Operational Replacement]. TUCOR was behind our lines in Sicily. Now and then there, you could hear cannon fire from us and the enemy."

During World War II, TUCOR was a classification used by the U.S. Army to manage the assignments and deployments of military personnel and resources within different theaters of operation. The office helped organize and direct the flow of replacements and resources where they were needed most, depending on the strategic requirements of each theater. Since Henry was a lawyer—and there were few specific positions open in the Army for lawyers—the Army, at that moment, had no permanent place for Henry, the lawyer, so they essentially moved him into "Army limbo."

After being attached to TUCOR for a while and learning to shoot a .45 automatic ("I don't know what I would have done with it, but I learned how to shoot it"), Henry was shipped out to Italy, Headquarters, Second Corps, and was assigned as an adjutant to a general whose name he could not recall.

From this point forward, Henry starts writing numerous letters to his mother, father, relatives, and so on. Henry's letter writing is so fertile that at the war's end, he has written nearly 108,000 words between 1943 and 1945 when he was discharged.

Untypically, these letters from a soldier, an officer serving in various combat zones in and around Italy, Algeria, and Sicily, have very few words about combat, enemy soldiers, battles, or the devastation that the war brought to those theaters. Further, we have an atypical perspective of the combat zones Henry has passed through. This was fortunate for Henry because he was not getting shot at and didn't have to shoot anyone with a .45 that he barely knew how to handle.

Between 1943 and 1945, Henry wrote many letters through V-Mail.

During World War II, V-Mail (short for Victory Mail) was a mail process used to correspond with soldiers stationed overseas—also used by civilians back home writing to soldiers in the theaters of war. It was developed to conserve shipping space because sending traditional letters and packages required substantial cargo capacity that was better utilized for essential war supplies. Ordinary mail took up volumes of space and weight. V-Mail involved a specific process where written letters were converted into microfilm. These microfilms were then shipped to the recipient's country, reprinted on smaller-sized paper, and then delivered to the intended recipient. This system dramatically reduced the volume and weight of mail. V-Mail ensured that soldiers and their families could maintain communication, boosting morale while ingeniously and efficiently managing logistical challenges.

Of course, all V-Mail was censored. Anything sensitive regarding the soldier's position, organization, the village or cities he was in, as well as any other tell-tale signs, were redacted. Often, soldiers would include little clues regarding their locations. Henry was lucky—since he worked in offices, he almost always had access to typewriters which meant he could add more information to his letters than if handwritten.

Typically, at the beginning of each typewritten letter and to give the censor an idea that he has not included sensitive items in his letter, Henry would type:

Censored – Henry C. Lowenhaupt, 2d Lt. AGD

In one letter, Henry gives a clear indication of the censorship his letters were up against. In one, he types: I wish it were possible to follow the channels of communication to have Barney find me if he comes here but I cannot give my address to you to give to him.

The government provided postage-free stationery in the shape of a cross. After typing on the empty spaces, the sender conveniently folded the cross into the shape of a letter with a place for the recipient's address and the postmark.

Sending letters outside the V-Mail system, while possible, would have been less efficient and potentially riskier both in terms of personal security and the likelihood of the letter reaching its destination. Regular mail did not have the same level of security and censorship as V-Mail, which was designed to prevent sensitive information from potentially falling into enemy hands. Letters sent via the regular post were still subject to censorship but were less secure and had a higher chance of being intercepted.

V-Mail streamlined the delivery process by reducing the physical bulk of mail, allowing more letters to be shipped faster, being lost or destroyed due to transport issues, military actions, or logistical errors.

Thus, we have little indication of the geographical location Henry writes about, aside from occasional broad strokes. Too often, detective work is insufficient to determine what village or town Henry is located in, and we are charged instead to filling in the blanks ourselves.

Often, aside from the V-Mail restriction, we wonder how much of Henry's discretion forces him to keep a top-secret oath regarding the work he does.

Henry graduated from Harvard College and Harvard Law School—and we sense this through his finely crafted, thoughtful, often serious typewritten observations. At Harvard, he learned to be a polished writer, an observer, and a recorder of the particulars that others might have shunned.

We see in Henry's letters how he found friends wherever he went, his love of the classics and Latin and St. Augustine, his passion for music and piano, his attraction to fine crafts and artisans, and his obsession with food, particularly local food. His sense of humor also comes through these letters. We see the dedication and love he had for his mother and father and the others in his family. You will find names of friends—both from St. Louis, where Henry was born and raised, and newly found friends he made among local people and the military wherever he was stationed. Some friendships lasted throughout his life. Others are lost in history.

While Kesselring and von Richthofen were planning and devising complicated strategies to win the war for Germany and outwit the Allies, Henry's intelligent observations show the reality of war-torn Italy at ground level.

And so, through Henry Cronbach Lowenhaupt's writings, we see in this narrative the horrors of war and the everyday minutiae that Italians had to endure.

It is a story of balance and a paradox of wartime Bari.

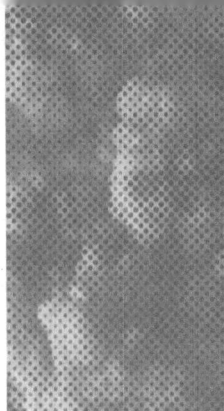

4

"THE SWEDISH TURNIP"

Before the SS *John Harvey* docked, the crew had been enduring days that merchant seaman dread. Since the *Harvey* had to wait five days for dockside unloading, the merchant seamen on board had little work besides the boring maintenance of their ship. Half took shore leave; all wanted to be back in the United States in time for Christmas.

The *Harvey's* skipper, Captain Elwin Knowles, made many trips to the War Shipping Administration office at the Stazione Marittima in attempts to get the ship dockside space to unload their hazardous cargo; his efforts did nothing to move up the shipping date, and the *Harvey* remained becalmed. When Knowles met with the British Port director, he was on the verge of telling him about the mustard gas to underscore his urgency—but Knowles was not supposed to officially know about his dangerous cargo;

it was top-secret. In fact, the Big Three—Roosevelt, Eisenhower, and Churchill— required a memorandum of understanding that the mustard gas was designated top secret. The transportation of mustard gas aboard a ship into Bari, a war zone, was also top secret. Only a handful of people aboard the *Harvey* knew what was under their feet. And if Knowles told anyone, trouble would follow that would be seriously unfavorable to his career.

Earlier, when Knowles' fifteen-ship convoy entered the breakwater outside the harbor at Bari, they had to pass through the submarine nets between the Molo Nuovo and Molo San Cataldo. When they did, Knowles shook his head in irritation when he saw the condition of the harbor; he picked up his binoculars. His vision only magnified his frustration. Everywhere he looked—along the two moles he had just passed, along the shorter Molo Pizzoli, the Molo San Vito, and Molo Foraneo—merchant ships were anchored at every nook and cleft—like babies lined up in the nursery. No room at the inn. Knowles forced now to anchor the *Harvey* along the already crowded East Jetty.

A man who had to know about the mustard gas was Lt. Thomas H. Richardson, *Harvey's* cargo security officer—a bundle of nerves by mid-afternoon on 2 December. He also had done everything he could to get the mustard gas offloaded: contacted every military officer at the port. Felt he could do no more. Both officers were at an impasse.

Standing on *Harvey's* bow, Richardson stared at the charming city, the puffy clouds.

Imagined the SS *John Harvey* was asking for trouble just sitting here like a fat goose.

And with all that mustard gas below deck.

Knew, too, that the harbor—Bari, beautiful Bari—was not nearly prepared to defend itself effectively.

Knowles stood beside Richardson in silence.

Then, "*Look!*" Richardson shouted.

Above, a lone plane—looked like an Me 210—scribing a fast line over the harbor. Richardson wondering if the crew on the aircraft could see the ships below could count their numbers. Record their names? Why would a single Luftwaffe plane fly over Bari unless it was on a reconnaissance mission? Prelude to an attack? Why couldn't complacent officers back at the War Shipping Administration office at the Stazione Marittima deduce this? An attack was inevitable, wasn't it? Complacency? Too many layers of bureaucracy? If they understood, they could have adjusted the offloading schedule and gotten things done faster. Or spread the ships out into the harbor instead of positioning them like eggs in an egg carton.

It was a reconnaissance plane; that's what it was.

Clear and simple.

And it was evaluating the harbor.

The ships

Your ship, Knowles!

Hauptmann Veit Renz and Dieter Jürgens certainly saw the merchant ships—all of them: counted them with uncertainty because Veit was flying the plane and Jürgens was busy with the camera. The Hag's vibrations, the jitter, stuff like that—27 or 30 ships.

Targets.

Renz and Jürgens had no idea about the mustard gas in the *Harvey*.

Then Renz crushed the throttle forward and was shooting back to his base in northern Italy. He knew once von Richthofen got his report, the pictures, the drawings, he'd launch the attack. Every minute, every second, the ships remained unopposed meant more supplies to the Allies.

Maybe a silver goblet, after all.

Generalfeldmarschall der Flieger von Richthofen waiting for him and Jürgens.

Hauptmann Veit Renz knew his field marshal. Knew his reputation. His proclivities.

Wolfram had a reputation for his technical expertise and detailed approach to military operations. He was deeply involved in the planning and execution of air strategies, demonstrating a keen analytical mind and applying this to what he hoped would be a memorable attack on Bari and all those merchant ships. At the same time, much like his cousin Manfred—the Red Baron—Wolfram was an ambitious and driven officer—and these traits drove his career and led him to become the youngest and shortest field marshal in the Luftwaffe, equivalent to a five-star general in the US army—no easy attainment. He was not averse to taking risks to achieve his objectives and always demanded lofty standards. Throughout his career, Wolfram showed his capacity to adapt to changing circumstances and technologies. Evident throughout various military campaigns, he could innovate the use of air power. Many would say, too, that Wolfram had gravitas; the short field marshal's presence was felt immediately when he strode rebar straight into a room, and you saw him the first time.

And always, he had a few special tricks up the sleeve of his bespoke field marshal's uniform.

One in particular that he ordered his pilots to utilize when bombing Bari: The wholly unorthodox "Swedish Turnip" (AKA Rutabaga) on the Bari attack.

In the earlier days of the Luftwaffe, fighter pilots quickly learned about what they called the Swedish Turnip. Since a Swedish turnip grows in the ground, the upper half presents a squat silhouette—the ship—thus, the name for the maneuver. They all recognized that the best approach to attacking a ship was abeam, not from high up in dive—but low, within feet of the water's surface. The closer the fighter flew above the water's surface, the higher the ship's silhouette resolved. Thus, a better chance of hitting the target. Through trial and error, the pilots found that this maneuver was best performed at dusk or in moonlit conditions when the camouflaged fighter's silhouette was thinner and harder to spot. But this took a lot of nerve. One such pilot was Wing Commander *Oberstleutenant* (Lieutenant Colonel) Robert Kowalewski, a Knight's Cross recipient, one of the few fighter pilots who had refined the Swedish Turnip—actually, one of the few who dared to do it.

Kowalewski approached his target, the ship, at 200 mph and an altitude of forty-five meters. This was difficult and dangerous, especially at dusk; most barometric altimeters were unreliable. Often, the pilot would not rely on or even glance at the altimeter because if he did, the altimeter would tell him he was flying several feet underwater—then he would be disoriented. Kowalewski had to fly perfectly level and at a precise altitude and speed—about 200 mph—avoiding his propeller tips from slicing into the water and the fighter nosing over into the sea and killing him. Kowalewski crafted meticulous calculations before he tried the maneuver the first time; he practiced this over and over a body of water. He estimated the speed and altitude of the bomb: After it was released from the aircraft, the bomb would fall five meters the first second, fifteen meters the second, and twenty-five meters the third, a total of forty-five meters. The bomb, meanwhile, flew straight and level for two hundred and forty meters, give or take a meter or two, before hitting the ship. After release, the first three seconds, the bomb's loss of momentum was minimal, and it flew along underneath the bomber. It lost inertia and slowed into a gentle arc toward the ship's gunwale (pronounced "gunnel").

Did it work?

In the early part of the war, *Oberleutenant* Kowalewski's Turnip maneuver proved perfect: He sank three ships using the Swedish Turnip all on one sortie. He is credited with sinking more than a hundred thousand tons of Allied shipping, and many others copied his method, but none achieved the numbers he did. By using the Swedish Turnip, Kowalewski did indeed deserve his Knight's Cross.

Of course, von Richthofen was aware of the Swedish Turnip and Kowalewski's prowess as an *experten* pilot. The field marshal strongly suggested that, if practical, some of the 109 Ju 88s use the Turnip to get under the radar at Bari and to reach the harbor before harbor defenses were initiated. And for scoring numerous direct hits on the anchored ships as they came in low and fast above the surface of the harbor.

Surprise number two from von Richthofen was chaff.

The Germans used the code word *Düppel*; the British dubbed it Window.

Most of von Richthofen's Ju 88s were equipped with

Düppel—thin strips of either aluminum, metalized glass fiber, or plastic. The *Düppel* version—the real McCoy and not a makeshift substitute—was a sheet of paper with tin foil pasted to one size—the kind you use in an oven. Many times, the Germans would print a message on the paper side for citizens to surrender and the tin foil on the reverse—two birds, one stone. A typical piece of *Düppel* measured almost eleven inches by less than an inch and was packed into bundles, each weighing one pound. Once dispersed, chaff produces a large radar cross-section, bright white on radar screens, intended to blind or disrupt radar systems and confuse them from detecting aircraft. On a radar screen = it looked like a Fourth of July explosion against the night sky. This made it difficult for the gunners on the ground to distinguish between an aircraft and thousands of strips of household tinfoil. This caused concern in RAF Fighter Command and Anti-Aircraft Command—they managed to suppress the use of Window until July 1943 for fear that once they started using it, the Germans would too. It was felt that the new generation of centimetric radars available to Fighter Command would cope with Luftwaffe retaliation. But the British could only hold out so long, tempted to grab an advantage, and used their Window on a bombing raid to Hamburg in July 1943; it surpassed expectations. British bombers' losses dropped nearly in half. Göring did not take long to realize the advantage of this and ordered his Luftwaffe bombers to use *Düppel* when suitable.

A large supply had been requisitioned and cut into thousands of strips to deceive flak gunners' radar installations along the Adriatic. Several other Ju 88s were designated to use parachute flares to light up the Bari harbor, giving pilots and navigators a more precise target for dropping their bombs.

While von Richthofen's bombers were warming their engine oil, waiting to take off on what promised to be a historical date, back home, US history was being written throughout this year.

In the United States, there was the usual wartime tension as people continued to live their lives unhindered by bombings and historic battles in their towns and villages and destroying their property.

President Roosevelt and Prime Minister Churchill conferred in January at Casablanca, discussing the "unconditional surrender of Germany, Italy, and Japan."

The cost of the war staggered everyone's imagination. World War I, which lasted less than two years, cost about $35,000,000,000. By mid-year 1943, World War II was costing $8,000,000,000 *per month*.

Chicagoans rode in a subway for the first time.

Frank Sinatra captivated bobbysoxers of both sexes. Thirty thousand of Sinatra's fans reacted so riotously during his appearance at the Paramount Theater in New York that a riot call was sent out. No less appealing was Dinah Shore, a dark-haired singer who charmed audiences with her rendition of *One Dozen Roses*.

Ayn Rand wrote the bestseller *The Fountainhead*. The other big book was *A Tree Grows in Brooklyn*.

The most popular shows on Broadway were *Oklahoma!* and *Ziegfeld Follies*.

In 1943, the average price of a movie ticket in the USA was about 29 cents. This period during World War II led to increased attendance at movie theaters as people sought entertainment and escape from the realities of the war.

Some of the popular films were *For Whom the Bell Tolls* with the handsome Gary Cooper and the stunning Ingrid Bergman; *This Gun for Hire* with Alan Ladd and *Watch on the Rhine*.

Popular movies in 1943 in Germany were *Münchhausen*, a lavish fantasy film made to celebrate the 25th anniversary of the UFA film studio, one of the major studios in Germany at the time. It was a technically advanced film about its era and featured Baron Munchausen's fantastical adventures. UFA would become a prominent studio in Weimar, Germany, known for producing a wide array of films, including notable works of German Expressionism. By 1943, UFA had been co-opted by the Nazi regime to produce films that aligned with their propaganda goals. The studio was under the control of the *Propagandaministerium* (Propaganda Ministry), headed by Joseph Goebbels. Films produced during this period were often designed to promote Nazi ideology, bolster the war effort, and depict the enemies of Nazi Germany in a negative light. Many of these films were characterized by their high production values and were used as tools for both domestic propaganda and international influence. Another film, *Immensee* (Immense), a romantic drama based on the novella by Theodor Storm, was part of the regime's attempt to promote traditional German values. And *Romanze in Moll* (Romance in a Minor Key), a drama film that was among the more subtle and artistically inclined productions of the time, featuring a tragic love story.

A variety of radio shows captivated listeners across the United States, with genres ranging from dramas and comedies to news broadcasts and musical shows—all as popular as Netflix, etc., today. One of the most popular radio shows was *The Lone Ranger*. A Western adventure show first aired in 1933 that quickly became a hit with its tales of the masked hero and his sidekick,

Tonto. *The Shadow* is known for its famous line, "Who knows what evil lurks in the hearts of men? The Shadow knows!" This show thrilled audiences with its mysterious and suspenseful plots starting in 1937. *Fibber McGee and Molly*, premiering in 1935, this comedy show was beloved for its humorous look at married life and featured the famous "cluttered closet" gag. *Amos 'n' Andy*, starting as a radio serial in 1928, this show became one of the most popular and, later, controversial shows for its portrayal of African American characters by white actors. *War of the Worlds*. This 1938 broadcast by Orson Welles and the Mercury Theatre on the Air was famously mistaken for a real alien invasion by some listeners, illustrating the power and impact of radio.

Major radio networks then were NBC (National Broadcasting Company), CBS (Columbia Broadcasting System), ABC (American Broadcasting Company), and the Mutual Broadcasting System. These shows and networks played a pivotal role in shaping the early landscape of American entertainment and mass communication, making radio a centerpiece of American culture during its golden age.

People were listening on their radios to the most popular songs that year: *Besame Mucho—Kiss Me Much, Do Nothin' Till You Hear from Me*, and *Mairzy Doats* (Mares eat oats and does eat oats, a little lamb'll eat ivy).

And Henry Lowenhaupt, where do we find him and what keen observations do his letters convey about Italy, the Italians, the war?

While numerous writers, war correspondents, and pundits described in detail the landscape of war, perhaps none portrayed the ordinary challenges of everyday life of the Italian people as did Henry Lowenhaupt. He should have been writing for national magazines like *Life* or *National Geographic*, both established in 1943.

On November 27, 1943, days before the bombing, Henry wrote a long letter to his mother; we read what interested him at that time in his life in a battle zone. At the time he wrote this letter we deduce he was somewhere near Naples:

Dear mama –

Well – I suppose we should be thankful for one day of sun – as we had yesterday – Last night it started to rain again – and it is still raining. I suppose it will stop in about a month – meanwhile I shall quit writing about weather and mid – until I can say something nice about it. M Now I am mud-bound – just can't walk the mile to town, because it is knee-deep all the way.

I received three little volumes of Shakespeare from Ruth a few days ago – and last night read Measure for Measure with great pleasure. I think it shows Shakespeare just beginning – for here and there, a burst of great poetry comes through, and the ideas are beginning to appear tentatively, kind of experimentally, which later make the great passages of Merchant of Venice (Quality of Mercy) and Hamlet (about death). It is as if Shakespeare is trying a few of these thoughts to see if the audience will take them or fall asleep – and they make the play very interesting.

Other than that, not reading recently – a little of St. Augustine – who discusses a problem I must check in the King

James Version of the Bible. As a matter of arithmetic, he says the Hebrew Bible makes Methuselah survive the flood by 20 years – but says that only Noah and his three sons and their wives survived it. So I shall add up the ages and see how it works out in King James. Do you want to compare your Bible – the one said to be a more nearly literal translation?

Which reminds me of a passage in Cicero, which I cannot quote exactly – in praise of old age – He is refuting the proposition that old age is uncomfortable because death is closer. After denying the proposition, he goes on to compare death to quenching a fire. A great, roaring one can hardly be extinguished. And to plucking fruit – "If they are green, they can hardly be pulled from the tree; but when they are mature and ripe, they fall almost of their own weight." Contradicted by the bible – it took the great flood to extinguish old Methuselah – even though at almost a thousand years he must have been mature and ripe.

Love -
Henry

While Henry's letter is a well-written watercolor of his daily activities, people who are not family or friends might get the impression that Henry is not in the United States Army, not in a battle zone, or a soldier participant in the war. Because almost every letter contains no information about his observations or thoughts about his duties. Henry obviously did not have to worry about carrying or cleaning an M1 Garand rifle or sleeping in a trough of mud every night. Besides, Henry was fully aware of the restrictions placed on G.I.s regarding any kind of military details in letters home.

* * *

After Renz took his photographs and made drawings and flew off to report to von Richthofen, a tall, dark-haired British officer stepped out of the Office of Harbor Defense, looked up, and watched the contrails from Renz's Me 210.

Captain A.B. Jenks had the thankless duty of trying to organize a defense system for the harbor—a harbor controlled by several overlapping authorities. Of all the men assigned to duty at Bari, Jenks was the one man who knew he lacked enough of anything to put up a serious defense—not enough manpower, not enough proper weapons, and certainly not enough support for him and his efforts. When he spoke with the British military superior, he received a curt response. They told him that even if they did have enough materials, it really wasn't moot because British Air Marshall Coningham, commanding officer of the British air forces supporting the Eight Army, had held a press conference earlier today—hours before the attack—assuring everyone that the German Air Force in Italy had been thoroughly defeated; the Germans did not have the resources to intervene in Allied operations here in the Bari area. "I would regard it," Coningham had announced at his press conference, "as a personal affront and insult if the Luftwaffe would attempt any significant actions in this area."

Certainly not convinced, Jenks related the conversation to a fellow officer who laughed at him, saying, "The trouble with you,

Jenks, is that the Germans have you shaking in your boots. Ever since you lost your ship, you've been a pessimist."

Jenks had been assigned to a Q-class British destroyer shortly after the harbor had been opened. His task: sink enemy boats appearing along the heel of Italy.

Although Jenks' mission sounded significant, it wasn't—few enemy ships were sailing in the area. The most dangerous aspect of his mission was getting in and out of the Bari harbor and avoiding the mines the Italians had placed prior to surrendering, leaving them fused.

One morning, Jenks' destroyer was following three others into the port. The first three got in safely. Jenks's destroyer did not—it hit a mine.

Miraculously, Jenks' destroyer remained afloat; however, everything aft of the stern gun position was severely damaged, and thirty-two crew members were killed. Through his skill and seamanship, Jenks was able to maneuver his destroyer into a dock, but the ship was a total loss.

Standing here now with his fellow officer, Jenks acknowledged that this experience had made him desperately jumpy. Yet, he felt he had evidence to support his belief that the Germans were still capable of fighting back and attacking sleepy Bari. After all, Bari was lulled into complacency—the war was up north—and the Germans knew this.

And while the Allies wanted Bari left intact for their use, the citizens wanted their city untouched, not only for their safety but also for attracting tourism.

"THE SWEDISH TURNIP"

* * *

Sometime during Henry's exploratory walks and letter writing, von Richtofen was manipulating ideas for attacking Bari. Three approaches came to mind immediately and were presented in multiple briefing sessions.

Of the 109 Ju 88s assembled for the attack, several—the exact figure is unknown—were Pathfinders. It should be noted that that while 109 took off for the mission, 17 had to abort because of various reasons, leaving 92 to bomb and strafe the harbor.

Specially trained Pathfinder units were considered elite groups within all air forces—American, British, French, and German, and they underwent extensive training to perform their missions under challenging conditions. They were pivotal in maximizing the efficiency and effectiveness of aerial bombing campaigns throughout the war. Pathfinders were target-marking squadrons that located and marked targets with a variety of flares, red and white, at which a main bomber force flying behind them could aim, increasing the accuracy of their bombing. In the beginning of WWII, it soon became clear that bombs—particularly those dropped at night—had an erratic record of hitting their targets, that by the time the Luftwaffe, American or British bombers reached the target only one in 10 ever flew within five miles of its target. Half of all the bombs carried into combat and dropped fell harmlessly in open country killing trees and fields of hay and an unfortunate cow or two—unlike today's GPS-guided 99.5 percent accuracy. Only one percent of all the bombs were even in the vicinity of the target. Clearly something had to be done to address this, or some suggested the strategic campaign should simply be dropped; it was a waste of resources, and men were dying for nothing. Around this time Frederick Lindemann wrote an infamous report on "dehousing," (Dehousing was a strategy adopted by the British against the Germans during World War II. It looked to maximize the damage to civilian housing. The strategy was proposed via a memorandum on 30 March 30, 1942. Lindemann believed that this strategy would allow the British to avoid an invasion of Europe. After the Cabinet accepted it, it became known as the dehousing paper). It suggested that a bomber force be directed, focused, against German urban areas, destroying as many houses ("dehousing") as possible and thus rendering the German workforce unable to work well. While sounding good on paper, it was never met with a wholehearted reception.

While the Luftwaffe's Heinkel He 111 and the Dornier Do 217 were excellent Pathfinder aircraft, so was the versatile Junkers Ju 88—thus, von Richthofen had several assigned to act as Pathfinders on 2 December. These select aircraft would carry a payload of "marking ordnance" and light up Bari like a bright, sunny day. It is not known if these designated Pathfinders dropped parachute flares or, more likely, "flare bombs." A flare bomb hit the ground and ignited.

The ignition mechanism of a parachute flare typically involved a few key components that ensured the flare would ignite at the appropriate time after being dropped from the Ju 88s. A time delay fuse activated as soon as the flare was dropped and would light the ground below. This fuse was designed to give the flare enough time to reach a predetermined altitude before igniting—the flare would serve two purposes: it would light up the area below its descent and possibly cause fires when it hit the ground. The time delay allowed the flare to descend slightly after deployment but before ignition, maximizing the area of illumination from an optimal height. As soon as the time delay expired, the ignition charge within the flare would activate and ignite the main illuminating composition of the flare.

The primary chemical in the flare on this bombing run was magnesium, providing a bright white light. Magnesium is chosen for its high temperature and intense brightness when it burns. Also, oxidizers such as potassium nitrate or potassium perchlorate are used to supply the necessary oxygen for the magnesium to burn, especially since the reaction needs to sustain itself at high altitudes or in various atmospheric conditions where oxygen might be limited.

In the case of Bari and the altitude the Ju 88s would be flying, parachute deployment was almost simultaneous with the ignition of the flare. In some designs, the force of the ignition charge itself helped to eject the parachute, which then slowed the descent of the flare, prolonging its illumination time as it drifted downwards. The illuminating composition of the flare could be a mixture of metals like magnesium, which burns brightly, and other chemicals that determine the color of the flame. As the time delay fuse burns through, it ignites the main illuminating composition of the flare. The ignition not only initiates bright light but also generates gas pressure.

The parachute deployment, triggered by the increase in internal pressure from the ignited flare or a mechanical spring mechanism, triggers the release of the parachute. Once the parachute is deployed—manually through a chute in the plane—it blossoms and slows the descent of the flare. This allows the flare to illuminate a larger area for a longer period as it gently floats downward.

For the Bari mission, since the Ju 88s were flying over the harbor at about 800 feet less if flying the Swedish Turnip), the time after the flare was released to the time the parachute blossomed was minimal.

The area of light coverage by a parachute flare depends on several factors, including the flare's altitude, the brightness of its illumination, and environmental conditions such as weather or terrain. The intensity of the light produced depends largely on the chemical composition of the flare. Flares containing magnesium, for example, burn very brightly, enhancing the area of coverage. The brighter the flare, the further its light can reach, though this can also depend on atmospheric clarity, rain, fog, and snow, for example.

Typically, a well-deployed WWII German-manufactured parachute flare might illuminate an area with a radius of several hundred meters. Under ideal conditions, this can mean an area of over 100,000 square meters being lit up over the harbor at Bari, providing crucial visibility for the Ju 88s flying toward their targets—the laden merchant ships wallowing in the harbor.

Also, the higher the flare when it ignites, the wider the area it can potentially illuminate. The size of the parachute and the rate at which it descends influence how long the flare can illuminate an area. A slower descent prolongs the duration of illumination, allowing light to spread over a greater area as the flare drifts down.

The exact number of flares each Ju 88 carried to Bari—there were 109 on the raid—was dependent on the payload of the aircraft. Each model aircraft's payload was slightly different. For instance, how much did the bombs weigh?; how much gas was on board, etc.? All these factors would be subtracted from the gross payload number, then what was left was the amount of flares that could be carried—the more gas, the more bombs, the more ammunition, the less flares would be loaded.

Nevertheless, Bari's harbor, once the Ju 88s passed over, was going to light up with the spectral brightness of hundreds of suns, augmented by the brilliance from the explosions of the fuel and cargo aboard 27 merchant ships. A cauldron of hell it would be.

Further, there was a "bonus" attached to the flare drop for the German bombers—this was always the case when aircraft dropped flares. The flares would inevitably land on a structure, would still be burning, and cause fires, adding to the bombing destruction and sometimes causing more damage than the bombs that followed the flare drop. Leading up to the Japanese surrender in WWII, B-29 bombers were dropping a preponderance of flare bombs versus bombs or parachute flares onto Japanese cities. Since most structures were made of wood, vast sections of the city burnt down to ash in a matter of minutes. This also deliberately occurred numerous times in the bombing of Europe—in the case of the bombing of Dresden, burning more than half the city and causing 25,000 deaths over a three-day bombing run by British and American bombers within three months of the war's end.

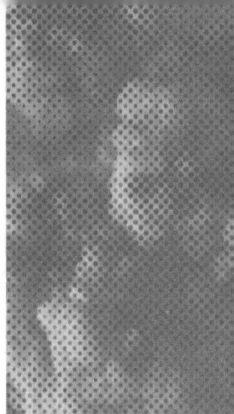

5

GENERAL JAMES HAROLD "JIMMY" DOOLITTLE

Until 2 Dec. 1943, Bari had been doing well. On 11 Sept., the Allies captured the city and placed it under the control and supervision of the British. Because of its strategic position—the harbor, mainly, was a major port supplying the Allies' northern advance in Italy. All the vitals of war were passing through: ammunition, food, parts, and gasoline, were going up north to supply General Doolittle's Fifteenth Air Force and the British Eighth Army.

Two days ago, Doolittle arrived in Bari and was in the process of setting up his headquarters. Days later, on 2 Dec., the Luftwaffe welcomed him to Bari. Most of the supplies in the harbor were for him, for his Fifteenth Air Force, and they were spread out among the Liberty ships Doolittle could see through his office window. Aside from the usual equipment were important medical supplies for the hospital units that the Americans and British were setting up to support the northern advance beyond the Gustav Line, a major German defensive line in Italy during World War II. Established in 1943, after the Allies invaded Italy, the Gustav Line stretched across the Italian peninsula from just north of Naples in the west, running through the Apennine Mountains to the Adriatic coast near Ortona. Natural geographic features anchored the line and were heavily fortified with gun positions, bunkers, and minefields. The most well-known and fiercely contested battle along the Gustav Line was the Battle of Monte Cassino—in fact, throughout WWII. Founded by St. Benedict in 529 AD, it is one of the oldest monastic institutions in the Christian world and has been a center of scholarship and religion throughout its history. At the time, it held some of the most valuable artwork in the world.

During World War II, the Battle of Monte Casino was a key part of the Italian Campaign, aimed at breaking through the Winter Line and reaching Rome. The battle involved several assaults between January and May 1944. Many Allied troops, including forces from the United States, Britain, Canada, New Zealand, India, Poland, and France, fought against the German defenders. The abbey itself was reluctantly bombed and destroyed by Allied forces in an attempt to dislodge a tenacious group of German troops, mostly *Fallschirmjägers* (paratroops), under the mistaken belief that the Germans were using it as a defensive position. The site was completely rebuilt after the war and continues to be an active Benedictine monastery, as well as a place of pilgrimage and historical interest. This series of four battles, taking place between January and May 1944, involved repeated and costly attempts by the Allies to break through the line and advance toward Rome. The monastery at Monte Cassino was used as an observation post—and was bombed and destroyed, yet the German defense remained resilient until the line was finally broken in May 1944. The Gustav Line's effectiveness was due to the challenging terrain and the strong defenses, which made it one of the most difficult barriers faced by the Allies in the European theater of the war.

The Allied forces involved were multinational, including British, American, French, Polish, Canadian, New Zealand, Indian, and other troops. The estimates of Allied casualties vary but generally include approximately 55,000 Allied troops. About 8,600 killed. Thirty-eight hundred were wounded, and nearly 8,400 missing or captured. German casualties were even more staggering. German troops from the 1st Parachute Division (*1. Fallschirmjäger-Division*) along with Wehrmacht and Waffen-SS units were killed and wounded in massive numbers—estimated between 20,000 to 25,000 (exact breakdowns are difficult to specify) and the number captured also hard to itemize.

Despite this, General Eisenhower felt confident about capturing Rome—the Allies' main objective—providing the weather didn't interfere. (Eisenhower did capture Rome on 24 May 1944, after one of the most difficult battles of WWII—the Battle of Monte Cassino.)

In March, Doolittle was elevated to commanding general of the Northwest African Strategic Forces, a position he held until 1 Nov. 1943, when the Fifteenth Air Force was formed and operated from Italian air bases in and around Foggi On 1 Dec.,

Doolittle called Bruce Johnson, his commandant, into his office in Bari and told him he wanted his whole staff moved to Bari. That consisted of two hundred officers, fifty-two civilian technicians, and several hundred enlisted men—and there wasn't a place prepared for their arrival.

While Doolittle was sipping his third cup of Joe and supervising the transfer of personnel, outside his window things were frenetic in the harbor. However, along the streets on the waterfront, life moved as it would have any other early evening, oblivious to the war's excruciations and the pending bombing minutes away. Bars and restaurants were doing their usual business. All the tables in the Hotel Albergo Oriente were glass-fronted and located on the lovely Corso Cavour, a wide boulevard in the heart of Bari with lilting palm trees; the hotel is still there today after a long and careful restoration. Blackout orders were suspended and the harbor was lit up all night—a beacon, a come-hither glare daring the devil to strike.

And not far away, on the waterfront of Porto Vecchio atop the roof of the empty Art Nouveau Margherita Theater, the radar installation that controlled Bari's antiaircraft guns was still being worked over. The gun crews had no warning of the German attack, and the guns were fallow throughout the raid.

At the time of the attack, Bari was packed with Allied shipping, including vessels carrying classified cargoes. The Allied commanders had implemented strict secrecy regarding the port's activities and its defensive capabilities. There were concerns that any defensive fire might accidentally hit other Allied ships or reveal the port's defensive capabilities and the types of cargo present to enemy aircraft.

The presence of ships loaded with ammunition and other volatile supplies made the use of defensive weaponry risky. The commanders feared that firing antiaircraft weapons could trigger falling debris from destroyed aircraft.

And, too, there was also a lack of coordinated defensive protocols in place at Bari at that time. The suddenness of the attack and the darkness may have also contributed to a delay in opening fire.

As a result of these factors, there was a delayed response in firing at the German bombers. Unfortunately, this contributed to the heavy damage and high casualties suffered during the raid. The raid exposed the vulnerability of Allied shipping concentrated in Mediterranean ports and led to changes in how Allied naval and air forces defended such critical supply hubs.

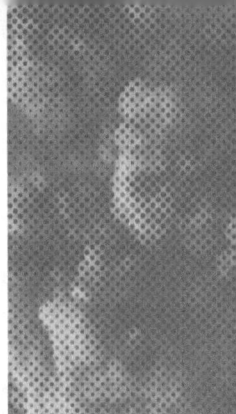

6

THE DEVIL IN MUFTI

The seaman aboard the ships in Bari's harbor, the people of Bari, the mothers, the fathers, the sisters, the daughters, the grandparents, will endure explosion and poison, impairment to limb and life, and at this moment will have no knowledge or can forecast what they will endure fully one hour from here when the insidious vapors from hell drape them, a horror they cannot defeat with weapon nor escape, but instead will remain victims in a landscape of ominous history.

The devil in mufti and with a *nom de guerre* that none know now and none will ever want to recall.

But someday, they will come to fathom the veil of gas, to despise it, dread it, and pray for its destruction and abandonment forever.

Several chemical signatures know the devil and do not care whose life it decays.

Organosulfur.

1,1-thiobis(2-chloroethane).

Dichloroethylene sulfide.

Yperite.

Iprit.

Bis(2-chloroethyl) sulfide.

$S(CH^2CH2Cl)^2$.

Eventually, mustard gas became an infamous name.

Despite these sing-song identities, mustard gas has no color—perhaps a light yellowish tint, if that. It is not akin to drizzle or light rain. Essentially, it is ghostlike, a haze—if that. Causes pain and death with the benign smell of garlic or horseradish.

When troops exchanged bullets and insults across the trenches in the Flanders vicinity in 1917 during WW1, they had no notion that their misery would be at least tenfold when the demon landed among them and that damned pervasive mud. This year, a new chemical would be introduced and weaponized, compounding their misery in "the war to end all wars."

The Germans that year, in their engineering zeal and quest for perfection in weaponry and munitions, let fly with a variety of shells containing the devil's gas: 155mm, 77mm, and 105mm shells, in addition to a variety of howitzers in interesting calibers and multi-colored circular markings, adding an extra band of suffering to "Dante's Inferno."

All shells were specifically tricked into dispersing mustard gas upon impact with planet Earth, oblivious to the ills she could concoct and let loose on humanity and then scatter or drift depending on the willy-nilly direction of the wind. The mustard gas bombs that rained down around Flanders contained liquid sulfur mustard or a thickened form of the agent. Think of it as a malicious liquid, gobby and gooey—particularly ugly because it *clings* to surfaces, like skin—and after exploding, designed to evolve magically into a haze hardly seen and scattered over a wide area after petting the ground. The impact will be extremely profound, utterly surprising, and artfully lethal, leading eventually to acute suffering and long-term casualties among soldiers and civilians and animals (both sides depended on horses and mules for conveyance, hauling guns and supplies; the animals screamed, too, don't forget. In fact, gas masks were custom-made and fitted to horses' heads; not so the forgotten mules). This gruesome legacy played a significant role in the development and signing of international treaties, such as the Geneva Protocol of 1925, which sought to ban the use of chemical and biological weapons in wars.

On 12 July 1917, down came a portentous variety of more than 50,000 artillery shells containing a hellish amount of poison gas into the ill-prepared ranks of scruffy Brits and Canadian troops fighting the fight near Ypres. There, sitting chewing on their breakfast and sipping watery G. Washington's Refined Coffee, the air suddenly smelling of garlic, or is that horseradish I smell—they sensed both—and desecrates their morning repast. The entire sky suddenly stunk. The whole world stunk! It did not take more than a few moments for the troops to figure out that the odor was not the cook's distasteful doing.

Oh, no, brother, it did not.

Something more insidious had come their way.

The troops had become somewhat accustomed to the widely

used chlorine or phosgene agents, which attacked the eyes and lungs—but this new terror burned their bodies both inside and out. Initially, the yellowish vapor did not give away its lethality, its nasty bite. But soon, yes, soon, the gas's toxic effect—it took about eight hours—would be upon them, and the troopers, they had no idea that they had been had—by German chemists' ingenuity and this deadly new invasion interrupting their morning calories.

But how could that be? How could garlic, delicious, ubiquitous garlic, be so hurtful and hate so effectively?

How?

Nearly 100 of the casualties succumbed to their deadly wounds within a few days.

Over the next several weeks, one million mustard gas shells were chambered into stout German cannons that would thump on Allied mud and young men near the lovely Ypres, leaving thousands writhing in anguish, disfigured, and, of course, unfit for duty. Recorded: 500 deaths.

Up and down the ragged front line, dressing stations overflowed with more than 2,000 victims writhing in pain from excruciating and untreatable blisters—a hundred times worse than blisters at the beach from too much sun but appearing just as virulent. Many soldiers had been almost immediately blinded while others started to slowly suffocate, to wheeze and regurgitate, because the gas was blistering and bleeding their lungs and windpipes. Suffocating, gagging, bleeding—an inimitable wounding had come to the battlefield, a new introduction to humanity's ability to bundle misery upon itself had visited the boys of WWI doing their duty on a battlefield already overflowing with pain and tenacious mud.

By the time they struggled to bring cheer that year, the use of mustard gas was *de rigueur* by all armies—including the holier-than-thou American army.

After entering the war in 1917, the United States could not resist and developed its nasty chemical warfare capabilities, including production facilities devoted to concocting mustard gas—the US Army deployed mustard gas in several engagements during the final months of the war in 1918.

Eventually, mustard gas became one of the most powerful tokens of trench warfare in WWI.

And, no, gas masks and respirators were not totally effective; they only protected the lungs, face, and eyes from the contaminant, and everything else burned crispy and pus-like, even skin covered by polluted uniforms. Too many troops hated lugging their gas masks from there to here. And too many of them, when they did put the mask on, felt claustrophobic. Boys wearing eyeglasses had a problem also—the mask did not fit them properly so they were abandoned.

Once detonated across a battlefield, sulfur mustard could take days to dissipate. Vapors, since they were heavier than air, would settle eerily into shell holes, craters, and trenches and taint the water that collected in No Man's Land. Men frequently, unknowingly, tracked poisonous mud back into their dugouts and bunkers before going to sleep, unwittingly tainting themselves and their comrades while they napped. According to one estimate, the British army alone suffered 20,000 mustard gas casualties in just the last year of WWI, 1918.

Unquestionably, this tit-for-tat use during WWI prompted the United States to secretly concoct and stockpile mustard gas throughout Europe—just in case the Germans forgot the past. They went flooey and decided to repeat the horrors. This time, if an attack occurred, the US would be prepared to kill, wound, and maim with its stockpiles of a devastating weapon that smelled like something you put in your spaghetti.

Thus, the reason for the secrecy of 2,000 mustard gas bombs aboard the SS *John Harvey* now looking for a spot to berth and unload its hazard and be off on its way for another boatload of supplies. It was, we assume, one reason for Churchill to withhold the truth: the knowledge that mustard gas had caused so much horror in WWI would have, he felt, created a massive panic—one more problem the prime minister did not need.

The last known large-scale use of mustard gas after Bari occurred during the Iran-Iraq War (1980 to 1988). Iraq, under the regime of the particularly repugnant Saddam Hussein, Chairman of the Revolutionary Command Council, and in complete disregard of the Geneva Protocol of 1925, used mustard gas and other chemical weapons extensively against Iranian forces and even against his *own* Kurdish population, most infamously in the Halabja attack in 1988. Saddam, in his bughouse brain, reached out for the most malicious, painful means to heap upon his enemy *de Jou*. This execrable overreach led to significant international condemnation, but since then, instances of mustard gas implementation have been reported in smaller-scale conflicts.

Initial gas effects are not confined to the skin or eyes: Victims can experience convulsions, dizziness, anorexia, and vomiting. Chronic toxicity includes debility, decreased vitality, attention deficit, increased sensibility, impotence, and cardiac autonomic abnormalities. An affected individual can experience a headache of varying degrees, anxiety, fear of the future, restlessness, confusion, and lethargy in mild and nonspecific neurological manifestations.

Victims will have to be transferred to a safe area as soon as possible—not easy to do in Bari where, after the bombing, half the city was torn to pieces and its peacefulness tossed aside. In the case of the bombing at Bari, this will be very difficult because of the number of victims and a lack of understanding of their malaise and the application of appropriate treatment. All victims' clothes will have to be removed, discarded, and burned. The skin will have to be rinsed with tap water and neutral soap. Rubbing and dry cleaning the skin will only increase the penetration of sulfur mustard into the victim's bloodstream. Eyes will need to be washed with large volumes of water, normal saline or ringer solution. Then, the victims should be transferred to a medical center or hospital for further medical monitoring. All the while hearing screams of excruciating pain.

Mustard gas continues to harm to this day. Abandoned stockpiles of the agent are frequently discovered and often injure those who stumble across it. In 2002, archeologists disturbed a lost consignment of mustard gas while performing an excavation at the Presidio in San Francisco. In 2010, a fishing trawler inadvertently dredged up some vintage gas shells from the bottom of the Atlantic off New York. Several of the crew were burned by the toxin and hospitalized.

* * *

Aboard the SS *John S. Harvey* at this moment, 2,000 M47 bombs. AKA "the chemical bomb." Each weighing about one hundred pounds or so—each containing filler, the "horseradish."

The chemical bomb was designed by the US military just before the onset of WWII to carry white phosphorus, jellied gasoline, or mustard gas, often referred to as the M47. The bombs aboard the *Harvey* are packed with mustard gas—also, in military terms, referred to as a "filler." The filler in military terms is known more kindly as the payload.

The design of the M47 bomb included a 1/32nd inch thin-walled, "burster-type shell casing," designed to splinter open upon impact when the powder charge went off and dispelled the chemical agent it carried. The gas is classified as a "cytotoxic" agent, meaning that it attacks all living cells it comes into contact with. Made of sulfur dichloride and ethylene, the thick, oily, brown liquid inside the M47 was intended to be delivered from aircraft, providing a convenient method for reducing the operational capabilities of enemy forces through contamination and injury. No need to unnecessarily jeopardize troops in hand-to-hand combat when you have poison on hand.

Visually—because Americans seem to think in almost all matters that bigger is better—the M4 chemical bomb was not massive—it did big things, but it was not *big* the way Americans might think in terms of SUVs and homes. Eight inches in diameter, forty-five inches from nose to tail, and weighing less than a hundred pounds.

The interior, looking at a cutaway of the shell, is filled with about 70 pounds of mustard gas, the payload similar to the viscosity of engine oil and yellowish. Passing through the center of the cylinder, a tube of "burster"—a black powder charge designed to explode and disperse the mustard gas. The burster in the M47 explodes on impact initiated by a fuse in the nose, causing the mustard gas to explode, achieving the intended poisonous effect.

* * *

The Ju 88s setting off to bomb Bari could carry a mixture of bomb payloads, depending on the mission. The Ju 88s on this mission could typically carry up to 6,614 lbs. both internally and hanging from the underwing racks. The bombs will range from 60 kg to 500 kg and, possibly but unlikely, 1000 pounds.

While not verifiable, the Ju 88s on the Bari raid more than likely carried several small bombs to maximize damage over a wide area—typical of an air raid designed to disrupt port operations. The exact number of bombs each Ju 88 carried for this mission would vary from bomber to bomber. Still, it is estimated that they carried a mixture of bombs (usually several 50 kg and 250 kg bombs) to inflict widespread damage on the harbor and ships— the smaller the bomb weight-wise, the more could be carried aboard a Ju 88.

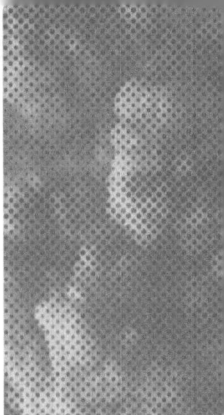

1

A WELTER OF SURPRISE

As bombing missions go, the Luftwaffe's bombing run to Bari and back to their bases would not be unusually elaborate, nor would it be too dangerous. Bari, after all, had no defenses to speak of, and there were no fighters available to defend the harbor.

Each Ju 88 had a pilot responsible for flying the aircraft. A navigator/bombardier handling the navigation and operating the bombing equipment. A radio operator/gunner managing communications and operating defensive guns.

The flight engineer/gunner looked after the aircraft's mechanical systems and also manned defensive armaments. All know what they will be facing—and compared to other missions they've flown, they feel this might be a "milk run." They know they won't be bothered by American fighters busy escorting B-24s and B-17s flying into Germany on bombing runs. And

Bari, the Luftwaffe crews know, has no significant anti-aircraft guns available because the system is in disrepair. Besides, they know that a lethargy has gripped the city and that the war is being fought up north, not here.

Today, the number of Ju 88s that will fly to Bari will be approximately 109. No data is readily available that definitively states the exact number of German aircraft that will bomb Bari and its harbor on this date.

As explained previously, Luftwaffe *Generalleutnant* (Major General) Peltz, 29, the youngest general in the Luftwaffe, brought an abundant amount of knowledge, tactical know-how, and experience to the Bari mission. Notably, he instructed his pilots to fly the Swedish Turnip—because he was ordered to do this by Richthofen. This maneuver would bring the Ju 88s down to 100 feet at 200 mph—anything lower or faster could have the Ju 88s smashing into each other or crashing. Peltz also gave field orders to fly east out over the Adriatic from their bases, assemble, turn south, and come in over Bari from the east, low and fast (the Swedish Turnip). This pattern, Peltz believed, would confuse Bari's defenders who would be expecting attacks coming down from the north. He also ordered a massive amount of *Duppel* to be cut to the frequency of the Italian radar signal. One hour later, the Ju 88s were warming their engines and would soon take off on a mission that would put them in the history books. The mission would be a nexus of multiple elements converging at that moment—one of them totally unforeseeable.

In retrospect, there would be many ways to view the raid: how fortunate, how unforeseen, and, at the same time, how chance led to palliative care for people with cancer.

The overall plan for the Ju 88's formation going to Bari called for the entire group of 109 bombers to fly in three main *Gruppen* (several groups), numbering around 36-37 aircraft. Within each *Gruppe* (Group), *Staffel* and *Kette* (Chain) formations will be staggered to provide mutual support and reduce vulnerability to enemy fighters—which in the case of Bari will be non-existent. The *Staffel's* formation will span several hundred meters wide, and with multiple *Staffel*, the formation could stretch up to two to three kilometers wide. But they cannot remain in this configuration throughout the bombing run. The formation will be staggered both horizontally and vertically to avoid bombers flying directly above one another. In-depth, a formation of 109 Ju 88s could be spread over several kilometers, likely around three to four kilometers in length, to maintain proper spacing for safety and bombing accuracy.

Quite often, on missions with groups eventually conjoining, the most dangerous part of the mission would be the assemblage of the groups into a pre-planned formation at a predesignated altitude—this often took as much as an hour or more. Bombers from different groups assembled into one formation after takeoff through a combination of precise planning, synchronized timing, a designated assembly point, altitude separation, and coordinated navigation. The success of this complex operation relied on the skill and discipline of the aircrews, effective communication (both visual and limited radio communication), and thorough, rigorous training. These procedures allowed diverse bomber units—such as the *Staffels* to spread out in northern Italy—to merge seamlessly into a formidable aerial force capable of executing large-scale strategic missions.

But when the formation approaches Bari, it will have to reform, contract—no wider abreast than the span of ships in the harbor below, or the harbor itself—perhaps two to three Ju 88s flying abreast.

This formation will involve forming a trail or a closely spaced staggered formation to focus their bombing run over the ships.

This tighter formation will ensure that the Ju 88s bombs are concentrated over a specific target zone—primarily the ships. This will reduce the risk of bombs missing the target due to dispersion caused by wider formations. And, in a congested airspace, what will form over Bari's harbor will be a streamlined formation that will prevent bombs from one aircraft falling onto an aircraft below. At the same time, a wider formation offers better defensive coverage en route; the priority over the target shifts to offensive effectiveness.

As they approach the enemy coastline and potential air defense zones, the Ju 88 formation will adjust altitude and spacing to mitigate anti-aircraft artillery effectiveness—which, in the case of Bari, the city, and the harbor, will be minimal.

The main focus will be to maintain formation integrity.

And it doesn't always work.

* * *

The history of bombing in WWII fills hundreds of books regarding Europe and the accuracy or inaccuracy of those bombing missions. The term "carpet bombing" emerged from WWII to cover the inaccuracy of falling bombs. Hypothetically, instead of bombing a single house with a single bomb, dozens of bombs were dropped, hoping for a hit. Despite the highly advanced

Norden and Sperry bombsights—advanced technology for the 1930s and 1940s—carried aboard the bombers, pinpoint accuracy was non-existent compared to today's laser-guided bombs and GPS technology. Thus, the B-17s and B-24s of WWII took a copious load of bombs up in the air stacked in their bomb bays. The more bombers, the more bombs that fell on targets. However, it was, essentially, a scattershot approach.

(The largest number of American bombers that participated in a single raid in Europe during World War II occurred on 3 February 1945, during the bombing of Berlin. On this date, over 1,400 heavy bombers, primarily B-17 Flying Fortresses and B-24 Liberators, were part of the raid. These bombers were accompanied by nearly 900 fighter planes, making it one of the largest and most powerful aerial attacks of the war—perhaps for all time.)

No single bomb and no single plane could have hit a target with one hundred percent accuracy under the conditions flown over Europe during WWII. Today's technology and its efficiencies had not arrived. As such, there were many trees, fields, and cows that got bombed and innocent people killed. And too, quite often, bombs were released indiscriminately when the weather was bad, or the bombers flew off target or suffered damage from flak or fighters. This, generally speaking, has come to be known as "collateral damage." It happens in almost every war and are generally facetiously referred to as Mistakes.

It will happen on 2 December in and around Bari.

Although the Luftwaffe that day had no intention of bombing Bari the city—its main target was the ships in Bari's harbor—they nevertheless unwittingly dropped a number of bombs on some of the most beautiful, historic sites in the world;

it was unavoidable. It would have been impractical and a waste of ordnance to bomb the city instead of the ships carrying war supplies to defeat the Germans.

The Ju 88s flying to Bari could carry up to 6,600 pounds of bombs internally and on external racks under their wings. Some later versions, especially those modified for long-range missions, might carry less depending on fuel loads.

So, 109 Ju 88s were flying the mission to Bari, each carrying 6,600 pounds of bombs—collectively, the force was carrying approximately 720,000 pounds of bombs.

Most of these bombs did effectively hit the main targets—the ships—but many would unintentionally hit peripheral buildings, streets, parks, etc., in the Old City (Vecchia) and the New City (Vecchi). As such, many merchant seamen were killed aboard ships in the harbor, as well as civilians in the area surrounding the harbor at the periphery of the explosions.

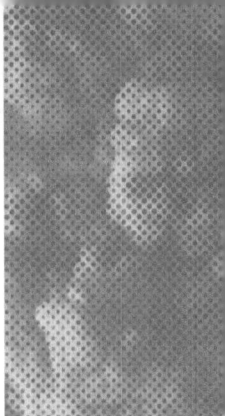

8

"CHE COSA?"

At 4:31 p.m., Bari's afternoon sun leaves the city alone with its hazards.

Throughout the frenetic harbor, the sun's flattery makes no distinction because it is brighter than a Christmas tree on fire. Not one light on ships, piers, and streets has stayed cold.

The thinking among citizens and military authorities is that the Germans are done picking targets like Bari—there are other richer, more crucial places to drop bombs, they believe. The Luftwaffe has insufficient crews, minimal amounts of flyable bombers, and few spare parts, and their gasoline reserves are paltry. Further, throughout Bari and the ships in the harbor, all have heard the regrettable words of British Air Marshal Sir Arthur Coningham, commander of the Northwest African Tactical Air Force, who mistakenly told the world that Bari was "immune from attack" from the Luftwaffe—giving himself high-praise for keeping Bari's sky "Luftwaffe free."

The attack will come later this evening. Conningham had precipitously and heedlessly announced that "the Royal Air Force had knocked out the Axis forces in the Mediterranean," injudiciously adding: "I would regard it as a personal affront and insult if the Luftwaffe should attempt any significant action in the area." The air marshal would achieve a dubious line or two in the history books with his precipitous words.

And so, Bari's hubris, its blatant overconfidence, was solidified to a fault.

With such words ringing in their ears, with urgency upon them to provide much-needed supplies to carry on the war up north, a total disregard to plan a substantive defense had been cast off with conceitedness.

How did this come to pass?

The harbor remained its own fool, weakened by a lack of planning and preparation for another bombing, an unprecedented, devastating bout—much like Pearl Harbor when the Japanese attacked with stunning astonishment. At the same time, soldiers and sailors that Sunday morning remained snug in their sacks asleep at the onset of the attack.

If General Doolittle's Fifteenth Air Force is going to do battle effectively again, it is best to leave the lights on tonight.

At this moment, Doolittle sits in a plush Art Deco office at the former Regia Aeronautica (Royal Italian Air Force) building on Via Napoli, a stone's throw from the harbor, the office known for its bold, geometric shapes and sleek, symmetrical designs

"CHE COSA?"

where generals and kings moaned about the war and dreaded its end and the treasures they had amassed.

Doolittle has read most of a debriefing report of a recent Eighth Air Force bombing mission. Simultaneously, he pushes away the empty plate of his evening meal at his desk. For dinner, he had *Bistecca alla Fiorentina* (steak Florentine style) served with broccoli rabe, sometimes referred to as "rapini," lathed with a tomato-based sauce that made his eyebrows arc. Then he finished a plate of recommended pasticciotto, a sweet treat from Pulia he had been told would make him moan, filled with custard and sometimes fruit or chocolate, popular for breakfast or as a dessert. He took a bottle of sparkling water served in a crystal glass with the meticulously engraved Regia Aeronautica logo, a bold eagle neatly rendered with outstretched wings, and no wine, thank you, because he needs a clear mind for the tasks ahead.

Jimmy Doolittle—a degree in aeronautical engineering from MIT—was renowned for his boldness, famously demonstrated in the "Doolittle Raid" during World War II, where he planned and led a daring attack on Tokyo in 1942. This mission required immense bravery, as it involved launching multiple bombers and crews from the USS *Hornet* a US Navy aircraft carrier—a feat never before attempted. For this stunning feat, Doolittle's nation awarded him the Medal of Honor. Doolittle, an aviation pioneer who made significant contributions to the development of aviation technology, including instrument flying in all weather conditions. He was not only a fighter but also an aviation pioneer. Doolittle made significant contributions to aviation, including instrument flying, which allowed pilots to fly in all weather conditions using instruments rather than visual cues.

His leadership style inspired confidence in his men because he was charismatic and able to inspire loyalty and bravery in those under his command. His courage and calm under pressure were qualities that made him a respected leader. A humble man, despite his achievements, known for focusing on the contributions of others. This combination of intellect, bravery, and leadership made him one of the most celebrated figures in American aviation history.

He stands now, wipes his lips, strides to the massive window, and looks out down Via Napoli, a mixed-use street, a vital vein for both residential life and commerce. While not overly abundant, there are a few green areas and small parks along or near the street, offering a respite from the stoney urban landscape. He notes, too, that the street houses several significant British and American military installations.

Glances down and checks his Army-issued Hamilton field watch.

7:23 in Bari.

Gives the crown a few quick twirls, back and forth, back and forth, to be sure it keeps running.

In the military, time, like oil and food, can be more vital than bullets.

The time you sleep, the time you wake, the time you fight, the time you die.

There is never enough, and the hands move fast or slow at their own pace.

Time is almost never a friend.

Because the hands never stop in your favor or theirs.

Just then, at this moment, this second, Luftwaffe *Oberleut-*

nant (First Lieutenant) Gustav Teuber, flight leader for *Operation Schuckert*, the force heading to bomb Bari, checks the Junghans clock on his instrument panel.

7:23.

Precisely.

Checks his caliber 40 twin-button Hanhart chronograph. Clocks in synch.

Fifty miles northeast of where General Doolittle stands pondering Via Napoli, the *Obereleutenant's* eyes stutter across the instrument panel below his windscreen: 500 feet above the Adriatic Sea and descending, heading west, speed 250 mph, oil temp good, fuel good. A lot of other details coming through the seat of his pants. As they do for all pilots. The Hag, surprisingly, feels strong. She looks at him in the eye: *Mir geht es gut,* ja? I'm doing good, right? The BMW 801 exhaust notes blistering the night air.

Then he presses the intercom button on the control yoke tied into the FuG -10 communications radio system and does a radio check with each crew member.

Josef Diefenthal, 23, observer/navigator/bombardier, an *Oberfeldwebel* (Sergeant Major) born October 2, 1920, Schalksmül, Westfalen, Germany.

Walter Drexler, 23, born March 3, 1920, radio operator/gunner, *Feldwebel* (Sergeant) from Mühlacker, Germany.

And Johannes Göhler, 25, flight engineer/mechanic/rear gunner. *Unteroffizier* (Corporal). Born 15 September, 1918, Bischofswerda, Sachsen, Germany. Göhler has the awkward position of lying on his belly facing rearward throughout the flight. Imagine that? Flying for hours like that in the Hag.

Oberfeldwebel Diefenthal will soon be the axis of the mission: The first man among the 109 Ju 88s to press the toggle switch and release their bomb load on the ships at the harbor. Not something Drexel feels comfortable with, this mass killing, no. Makes a promise to himself *never talk about this for the rest of your life.* This killing. Promise?

Diefenthal asking, "*Wie weit bis zum Ziel?*" How far to the target?

"*Achtzehn Minuten.*" Eighteen minutes.

"*Dank.*"

Then Diefenthal looks at his gloved hand.

Does not wonder why it is quivering.

* * *

Operation Schuckert held this formation out over the Adriatic Sea till now, reaching a pre-designated point directly east of Bari's beehive harbor. Now, thirty-five miles away from the target, *Oberleutnant* Teuber squints through the bug-smeared windscreen of his Ju 88 and sees the gleam of Bari's bright lights. They light up the whole universe! He does not have to see the silhouettes of the Ju 88s assigned duty as Pathfinders flying ahead; he knows they're out there, descending, coordinating their positions, and within a few minutes, will let loose with hundreds of parachute flares that will dangle and sway down—the glaring Christmas trees—and light up the city and harbor even brighter.

His breathing heavier.

Oberleutnant Fleich, flying thirty feet off Teuber's right wing, delicately tightens in closer to his squadron commander's Ju 88, the whole front line of their formation a treacherous wedge flying down to forty-five feet—the Swedish Turnip attack von Richthofen had prescribed. Although it is pitch black in the cockpit of Teuber's bomber, he dims the instrument panel lights, the better to see Bari looming ahead.

"*Lichter!*" Lights!

7:28.

Teuber recalling von Richthofen: "The Allies at Bari will keep all the harbor lights lit up because of the massive cargo that has to be unloaded as fast as possible."

But Teuber had been skeptical.

Wondering how the Allies, with so much precious cargo and so many brilliant tactical minds, could leave the harbor this bright at night, and be seen from many miles away—a true beacon, *please, come right this way!*

Now, he squints at the glow.

He can't believe it!

Never has he seen an enemy target lit this brilliantly.

Wie unverantwortlich!

How irresponsible!

But fortuitous!

This, he thinks, *Unter den Linden in Berlin on New Year's Eve.*

Yes!

He is at the forefront of the formation behind the Pathfinders, and if the Hag disagrees or is hit with groundfire or if a shell bursts nearby her careworn fuselage, she will whine and shutter and slide. Teuber hoping that she will hold her path.

He tightens his seatbelts. Sits up straight. Aiming for the light.

The harbor beckoning.

Teuber's ETA over the target: 7:30 pm.

* * *

Because the Allies planning the invasion of Italy wanted the city intact for their use after the landing, Bari was bypassed during the heavy bombardment phase that southern Italy had suffered.

Bari's old part, a labyrinth of alleyways, had been built on a peninsular cuddled by the Adriatic Sea on three sides. Composed of pleasant roads and charming squares bearing historical sites such as the Arch of Marvels, Basilica of San Nicola, Piazza Ferrarese, and Largo San Pietro—presenting, even in 1943, a medieval tone. Tonight, the old city, as usual, is crowded. The small side streets are playgrounds for kids, and soccer games are in progress on every block.

7:29 pm

Mass is scheduled for 7:30 this evening, and a small crowd meanders toward the church, worried they will not get a seat on an uncomfortable bench.

Many people hustle to Bambino Stadium to watch an American baseball game between two U.S. Army teams. The stadium situated in the northern part of the city near the Fiera del Levante area, not far from the Adriatic coast. Originally known as *Campo Sportivo del Littorio* when it was built during the Fascist era. Although it no longer exists today, the stadium played an important role in the early development of sports culture in Bari, particularly football. The area has since been redeveloped, and the stadium remains a part of the city's sports history. At one point, it became commonly known as *Stadio dei Bambini* ("Children's Stadium") because it was often used for youth and school sports activities. However, some said that Italian dictator Benito Mussolini had built the stadium as a reward to the citizens for producing the most babies in a specified period.

Although the battlefront tonight lies 150 miles north of Bari, no one in the city seems to care about the proximity. Right now, shop windows are showing off fruits and cakes, bread, and other delicacies not seen before the start of the war. And, as for centuries, young couples stride arm-in-arm. Despite the winter air, even the ice cream vendors are doing a good winter's trade.

* * *

Almost 7:30 pm, and many people in Bari do not grasp the muted drone—off somewhere east over the Adriatic. Or is it coming from somewhere else and echoing off the buildings here in Bari? Sounds like a deep hum, a swarm of Murder Hornets.

This prompts a question: Are General Doolittle's Fifteenth Air Force bombers buzzing at night? Since when?

Doubtful.

Many people glance up. Catch some night stars in their eyes. The night sky clear. No formation of bombers they can see. But they are looking up or should they be looking *out* over the Adriatic off on the horizon?

None of them have heard of the Swedish Turnip.

The unloading at the docks continuing at an unusually brisk pace—not only because of the determination to get the supplies up north but to move the ships out of the harbor and allow replacement ships to move in and offload.

Hustle.

Hustle.

Hustle.

None of the men on the ships or the docks at this moment looked up at the far-off drone; they are heads down, busy hefting, manhandling, hoisting a variety of crucial cargos desperately needed in the north. If they had looked up, they would have seen von Richthofen's wasps humming south over the Adriatic Sea.

Heading toward them.

Toward Bari and the ships.

* * *

Two days ago, before the Ju 88 Pathfinders dropped their Christmas tree flares and *Duppel*, an Italian schooner 135 nautical miles away a Castellammare di Stabia on the western coast of Italy loaded with olive oil slipped its moorings at the port and headed to Bari.

In command of the schooner was Captain Michael A. Musmanno, a US naval officer, formerly on the staff of General Mark W. Clark, the youngest American general in U.S. history when he was promoted to the rank of four-star general at the age of 46. He was best known for his leadership in the Italian Campaign during World War II, commanding the Fifth Army and later the Fifteenth Army Group.

Musmanno, of Italian descent, earlier had wholeheartedly agreed with the inhabitants of the Castellammare area that their food was not palatable without delicious olive oil. Thus, Musmanno decided to make a quick PR trip to Bari and obtain an ample supply for the people of Castellammare. Merchant Francesco Merefredo had owned the schooner he was using; it had been raised from the bottom of the port of Castellammare

"CHE COSA?"

after being spitefully sunk by the Germans when they evacuated the peninsula ahead of the Allied advance weeks ago. Merefredo agreed with Musmanno: If you raise and repair the *Inaffondabile* (Unsinkable), you can use it now and then. Four crewmen raised the hull, calked the seams, set up the masts, and replaced the 125-horsepower diesel engine that the Germans had removed.

They then sailed down the craggy western coast of Bari, the straits of Messina, a narrow strait between the eastern tip of Sicily (Punta del Faro) and the western tip of Calabria (Punta Pezzo), then north to Brindisi.

Arriving at Bari at 8 am on 2 Dec., Captain Musmanno made contact with a few officers he knew and obtained a load of flavorsome olive oil. That afternoon, the olive oil was loaded onto the *Inaffondabile*. After, the crew dined at a restaurant in Bari and returned to the schooner. There, Musmanno made a check of the cargo: three hundred quintals (112 pounds) of delicious olive oil stored in careworn vats. As he did his enumeration on the schooner, he was intent on counting accurately and paid no mind to the bees droning in the distance that was growing louder—like so many others in Bari had heard.

The *Inaffondabil's* sails cuffed the afternoon wind, and the schooner slowly cut out of the Bari harbor for Castellammare with Musmanno dutifully at the helm.

Now, he had a craving for a sweet, reached into his pocket, took up a popular Mars Milky Bar he bought at the American PX, and peeled away the wrapping.

He stood leaning, one hand on the helm, the other holding the Milky Way, munching.

Then, Michael Musmanno feels something flutter against

his ear—*a large insect, Michael?* He whacks it. Watches it spiral off his shoulder, pinwheeling to the deck.

What?

Must be the wind blowing debris in from shore.

A second later, another piece taps his nose, and another says hello to his right shoulder.

Long strips, shimmering Christmasy silver in the menacing dusk.

Silvery ribbons of twirling, whirling tinfoil everywhere, descending.

Flittering.

Floating.

Snowflakes.

One of the seamen rushes to Musmanno with a fistful.

"*Che cosa?*"

Then Musmanno understands.

Oh, he sure does.

Not insects, are they, Michael?

Duppel!

Michael knows!

"**Stop the engine! Spegnere il motore! Fermate, fermate!**" he screams. "**It's from a German plane. Get down!**"

Several Pathfinders crease overhead, their engines shrieking an extreme menace.

He dives and lands between two quintals, arms over his head, eyes shut.

Waiting.

Oberleutenant Teuber and the Ju 88s skimming the Adriatic Sea.

Lining up that Swedish Turnip.

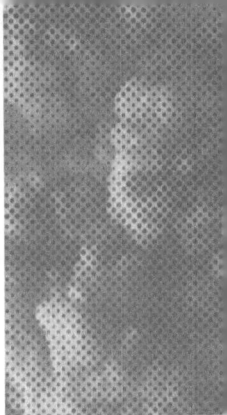

9

"I SMELL GARLIC."

Oberleutenant Teuber's POV:

Bari's lights glow brighter, larger, the harbor a dome of intensity.

Behind Teuber, a flank of Ju 88 bombers. Some in the leading edge formations dropping flares and *Tuppel*.

Teuber at 45 feet above the unforgiving Adriatic.

Skimming the black sea, heading for his target, the ships in the harbor.

Feeling that turmoil in his stomach.

"*Öffne die Bombenschächte!*"

Open the bomb bay doors.

"*Das Flugzeug gehört Ihnen,*" says Diefenthal, telling Teuber he has command of their plane until their bombs are away.

Oberfeldwebel Diefenthal's shaking finger flips a switch, and a rush of chilly air blows through the bomb bay.

Now, through Teuber's windscreen, down float the parachute flares from several Ju 88s stacked ahead, leading the group, the Pathfinders, delicate chandeliers swinging and swaying, descending into the target below, adding their light to the light, further lighting the target. Showing the way.

For the people on the ground, the first sign of imminent trouble is the rumbling sound, now a growl, coming from east of the harbor. For many, the sound is familiar.

Then, the flares. Not familiar.

Seconds after, *Tuppel* flutters down. A few moments later, tongues of anti-aircraft fire light up from the ships in the harbor despite orders to keep silent, bright red tracer lines scribing their ascent. This will not last long.

Diefenthal's eye peers through the reticle of the Lofte 7 bombsight, the standard in most German medium bombers during World War II. The Lotfe 7 series a precision bombsight designed for horizontal bombing and enabled accurate targeting from medium and high altitudes.

As a gyroscopic bombsight, it allowed greater accuracy in horizontal bombing. The bombsight had an advanced stabilization system to correct the movement of the aircraft and detect the wind's tendency, which improved bombing accuracy, and what the bombardiers loved was its simplicity and, in the right hands, effectiveness. On some Ju 88 models, the bombsight could be integrated with the aircraft's autopilot system, which allowed the plane to maintain a steady course during the bombing run, further improving accuracy.

Diefenthal saying, "*Bomben los!*"

Bombs away!

"I SMELL GARLIC."

Tonight, not all the Ju 88s carry the same bomb load, the same type; they bear a variety consigned for different purposes.

Aboard Teuber's bomber, SC Series High-Explosive bombs in an assortment of sizes from 50 kg to 500 kg. The tools of the ministry. The preacher's devil from heaven. The instruments of the surgeon. Also, an excellent choice for tonight is the SD Series Armor-Piercing bomb used for hardened structures and ships. Many of the Ju 88s have incendiary bombs (*Brandbomben*) and anti-ship bombs, such as the PC 1000 Armor-Piercing Bomb, designed to penetrate a ship's deck or hull and then explode inside the ship.

The first ship in the harbor to get slammed tonight, the SS *Joeseph Wheeler*.

For a moment in his office, staring out the window, General Doolittle has no idea what the hell just happened. He is shocked.

He turns, and a moment before he takes his first step, his office brightens blueish-white.

A million suns.

Maybe the electricity in the…?

What the…?

Then, a massive concussion. Doolittle stares out the window facing the harbor.

Towers of flame, columns of black oily smoke rising from the ships, and tracer fire reaching for harbor targets through the darkness. The general, slack-jawed, looking at a historic catastrophe.

An experienced officer, Doolittle, moves from his chair to the window. Then is slammed down on the floor. He tries to get to his feet, and a second concussion jolts him back. All the windows in the office shattered in unison, a hail of glass snow, flying over his head and across the office. The door buckles and splinters and blows off its hinges and slip-slides across the polished wooden floor. One look out at the harbor is all he needs—Bari has begun to suffer.

Another and another massive explosion of fire and smoke, billowing and roiling, concussion rings waving out, waving back, and a thunderous pounding racket.

Suddenly, Doolittle's aide, Bruce Johnson, appears. Both move to the window and watch one of the ships blow apart, and pieces fly and flutter, disappearing into the bleak night sky.

There was nothing much else they could do.

They stood there.

Many of the pilots, bombardiers in the Ju 88s took credit for the bombing of the *John Wheeler* after the mission, but no one was, or ever will be, officially designated as the first Ju 88 to blow up the *Wheeler*; to this day there are arguments about this kudo.

The bomb, whatever type it was, pierced the deck through the No. 3 hatch, exploded with ferocity and massive flashes after penetrating the hull, and ignited a large cargo of ammunition that sent a geyser of flame and skyrocketing bullets into the night sky. The concussion lifted and jolted Teuber's aircraft, and he had to jerk back the yolk. A perfect strike. The explosion heard three miles away and shattering thousands of windows in Bari. A burning hulk is the *Wheeler*I resting on her port side. The only Armed Guard survivors were the officer and twelve men who fortuitously had taken liberty in the town. Fifteen Armed Guards were killed or missing, and 26 of the merchant crew were missing.

Veit Teuber and Diefenthal shouting, two soccer players

who had just scored the winning goal, naturally, thinking it was their bomb, their aircraft, that struck the first blow—Teuber the lead in the formation, after all. *Had to be us*! And he could see the conflagration, the fireball rising in his rear-view mirrors, a mushroom of horror. Realistically, there was no way for the *Oberleutnant* to really know it was their Ju 88. After his bombs were released, Teuber flew easterly over the Adriatic, then came around to a northwest heading back to his base, had a few beers and a lot of agitated discussion and hand flying regarding what he and the others thought would be, historically, one of the greatest air raids by German aircraft. But before this celebration, he had circed back and strafed the ships, the quays until his gunners had no ammunition left.

They would laugh and talk loudly until they learned that they bombed a ship containing mustard gas and would kill nearly 1,000 people—men, women, children, dogs, cats. And that gave them more than a moment to ponder the repulsive power at their hands. Because all of them recalled the horrors of Ypres and the muddy trenches and relentless screams

Oddly, while the bombing of Bari and the spread of the deadly mustard gas was one of the worst aerial bombings ever, the world knew little details in the immediate days—because Eisenhower, Churchill, and Montgomery wanted it kept secret.

Ensign Eugene J. Kuhn, NSNR, the commander of the Armed Guard unit on the Wheeler. After the bombing, he filed a confidential report to Captain H.W. Zirolli, U.S. Naval Liaison Officer in Taranto, Italy, on 6 December, regarding the *Wheeler's* demise. Here, an edited version:

Subject: Report of Bombing Attack at Bari Italy, on 2 December, 1943:

1. The SS Joesph Wheeler... suffered direct hits by enemy bombers which attacked the harbor of Bari, Italy, between approximately 1920 and 1940, 2 December, with the loss of all hands who were aboard at the time. Fifteen members of the Armed Guard Unit, who were aboard, are either missing or killed. No trace of either crew could be found at the hospitals in Bari on 3 December, the day following the bombing.

2. ... Apparently the attack came as a complete surprise, since the alarm[s] sounded almost simultaneously with the dropping of the first bombs.

3. With three members of the Armed Guard Unit who had apparently passed onto the dock area before the British officers began ordering the men to return to the city, we did what we could along the breakwater. One occasion we tended the stern lines of a small tanker in an effort to clear it from a ship burning alongside. However, the tanker swing into the blazing ship after we cleared its line, and it is not know whether the ship's officers were able to take it out into the harbor and extinguish the fires.

4. After it became apparent that we could do little else of use, we returned to the city where we stopped at the headquarters of the 15th United States Army Aair Force.

We were joined there by nine Navy gunner who had been turned back from the dock gates and the remainder of the merchant crew.

5. The following day, hospitals were check in an effort to learn where there were any survivors from the ship, None besides those of us who were ashore at the time of the attack could be located

6. Delay in transit was caused when the ship went aground during the night of 4 December, 1943.

7. As the Defender Passed out of the harbor of Bari, we passed with three hundred yards of the SS Joseph Wheel's berth and from what could be seen of the remains of the vessel, it appeared that thew ship was on its port side and that its starboard side had been blow almost entirely away

—Eugene J. Kuhn

Within a matter of moments, the second ship to get blasted was the SS *John L. Motley*. Moored on the East Jetty between two Liberty ships—*John Harvey* and the *John Bascom*—and four ships north of the *John Wheeler;* the *Motley's* cargo consisted of ammunition, cyanide, and high-octane gasoline. She had been moored astern to the jetty, her anchor holding her securely facing the harbor.

Shortly after the parachute flares started to swing and sway down onto the ships, no alarms sounded. Lack of coordination it was: There was also an absence of managed defensive protocols in place in and around Bari—perhaps because of a lack of resources. The suddenness of the attack and the darkness may have contributed to a delay in opening fire. And bombs from the Ju 88s were dropped before the shore batteries commenced firing; so, the Ju 88s passed over the harbor untouched—or, at least, most of them did. The ground fire was minimal and ineffective.

Luckily, none of the crew of the *Motley* were on board their ship—and not much of what specifically occurred in the *Motley* is known. However, an Armed Guard member aboard the adjacent ship, the SS *John Bascom*, stated that three bombs hit: one in number five hold, the second in number three hold, and a third went down the ship's smokestack. Further, he stated that after the number five hold was hit, fire broke out but was brought quickly under control. Last, when the number three hold caught fire, the crew was unable to extinguish it.

A witness stated that "as the attack began, the bright lights illuminating the piers and harbor were promptly extinguished [too late]—except for spotlights (or searchlights) situated on a shore crane. This crane was abandoned by panicky Italian personnel but the light remained on for about 9 minutes until shot out by British Military Police."

Undoubtedly, a beckoning beacon for the German pilots.

Cadet Leroy Heinse, a member of the *Bascom* crew, recalled what happened as soon as the parachute flares descended: "they lit up the whole harbor. You could just sit there and read a book, so to speak, because of the brightness. Just about the time I was arriving in the wheelhouse, a bomb hit our ship just forward of

"I SMELL GARLIC."

the wheelhouse and it went into the hold. There was a tremendous explosion. It was so great that it blew off all my clothes. Shoes, everything. The only thing, to the best of my knowledge, was that I was left with were my dog tags and silver identification bracelet on my left arm."

A Navy gunner, Stanley Bishop, gave a graphic statement to the Associated Press:

I was sitting in the mess hall writing a letter home. All of a sudden the general alarm sounded, and the guns began to go off. I dopped y pen and tore up to the gun station on the bridge. The sky was full of of tracers and flares and exploding shells, and it looked just like the Fourth of July.

The first tick of bombs plunked about 100 yards away, striking nearby vessel which exploded and sank.

There was a heavy jar and a wave of heat. Then there were explosions all around us. The ship next to us was burning.

I got out about 400 rounds of 20-milimmeter gun before an erupted shell jammed it. Then two or three bombs hit our ship.

One bomb killed the man next to me and blew me off my feet. The air was full of flying splinters and stuff, and a couple of German planes were strafing.

After the ship was hit, I went below to help bring up the wounded. Practically everybody in the crew was either dazed or hurt bad.

Ensign Vesole was shot all to pieces and hardly able to stand up, but he was in control all the time. Reeling over the deck, he was giving orders and helping the wounded.

…I was hit in the head by shrapnel so much that my helmet was cut to pieces.

The harbor had turned accursed within a minute after Teuber's initial Ju 88s thundered over, dropping flares, Tupple, and their Whitman's variety of ordnance.

Most of the Luftwaffe pilots approached the ships in the harbor using the Swedish Turnip, despite the fact that many thought they would have to change their laundry after the first run. Most swung around and strafed everything—the ships, the quays, and the docks.

The concussions and explosions on and around the Bascom were ruthlessly strong, knocking men off their feet, piercing them with shrapnel. Every man aboard was peppered and punctured with steel the size of popcorn and watermelons. The shore batteries, silent, had no warning of the raid, so they did not load their breaches and fire at the most propitious time—before Mr. Devil pulled his gloves on.

According to the Italian Berthing Plan, the SS John Harvey was moored between two berths, 29 and 30, and the Motley to her starboard side. A nearby ship exploded and showered flaming debris onto Harvey's susceptible decks. Many of her crew were ashore on liberty at the onset of the attack. Her complement was 40 crew members, 28 Naval Armed Guard, and 10 U.S. Army Chemical Warfare personnel. However, soon after the raid started, only seven of the eight passengers were aboard. The six merchant crew and a U.S. Marchant Marine cadet that were ashore were the only survivors.

The SS John Harvey was at the core of the mayhem at Bari—aside from the 109 Ju 88s bombing and machine-gunning the ships and their massive bomb load loosed over the harbor at 7:30 p.m.

The Harvey had been bearing a secret cargo: 2,000 meticulously and oh-so-carefully assembled American manufactured M47A1 mustard gas bombs, each containing 60–70 pounds of the agent. According to Royal Navy historian Stephen Roskill, the *Harvey* sailed to Europe with mustard gas for *potential* retaliation against Germany because of an alleged threat to initiate chemical warfare in Italy; this threat was stillborn.

Harvey never got a chance to fire her guns. Her armament was stern-mounted, a 4-inch (100 mm) deck gun primarily for use against surfaced submarines. Totally ineffective regarding the Ju 88s flying overhead at over 200 mph.

Built by the North Carolina Shipbuilding Company in Wilmington, North Carolina, she was launched on 9 January 1943. Her Maritime Commission Hull Number was 878, and she was rated as capable of carrying 504 soldiers.

It is impossible to tell the trajectory, the exact Ju 88, the exact type of bomb, and the type of initial destruction that flipped the switch on the catastrophic chain of explosions releasing the gas. It is also impossible to tell if a single bomb hit the *Harvey* at a single moment, pierced the decking, and then exploded below deck—if so, a most fortunate occurrence for the Germans. The odds are good that the bomb was a PC 1000 Armor-Piercing Bomb. The Germans certainly and deliberately included this type of bomb in their shopping list prior to take off—armor-piercing—knowing that many non-piercing bombs detonated on ships' steel decks and hulls; the plan was to get bombs *inside* the ships' hulls where the ammunition and gasoline were stored; secondary explosions are most effective for demolishing objects such as ships, trains, and tanks. Many *Deutschewerke* bombs tonight achieved that objective. Many. A nanosecond into the hold of the ship, the explosion from the PC 1000 Armor-Piercing

Bomb wracked ammunition, bulged hulls, spread mustard gas, and anything volatile. It played no favorites. Some said that the force of *Harvey's* explosion was so fierce that the hull rose like a steel cadaver rising from the water a few feet, a colossus, and then pounding down mortally wounded and finally giving its soul to the harbor's depth and military history.

The explosion of *John Harvey* caused liquid sulfur mustard from the shattered bombs to spill onto harbor waters already contaminated by oil and flame. Many sailors who had abandoned their ships and jumped into the fiery water were going from "the frying pan into the fire"; their uniforms had become slathered with the oily mixture and greasy diesel fuel, which provided an ideal solvent for the sulfur mustard to cling to flesh and clothing. Some mustard gas mingled with the thick clouds of smoke and massive flames, indiscernible. And, its pernicious effect moved stealthily throughout the city of Bari, expanding its hellish specter across a landscape of American and British service members and then, *hello*, to hundreds of Italian civilians. The wounded seamen were pulled from the water and sent to medical facilities whose personnel were initially ignorant of mustard gas and its harmful effects. And so, too, the medical staff who focused on personnel with blast or fire injuries and little consideration given to those merely covered with oil. (It would take ten to fifteen minutes for the gas-inflicted skin to show signs of injury or pain.) Many injuries caused by prolonged exposure to low concentrations of mustard might have been reduced by bathing or a simple change of clothes.

Operatic was the scene in the harbor, in the city.

The bombing of *John Harvey* and the mustard gas was happenstance gone bizarre.

And overall, a carapace of political and military secrecy.

Instead, throughout the harbor the ships, and the city, panic was endemic.

No space, no cover, no area offered sanctuary. Not tonight.

No shelter existed.

There was no pause in the pain.

The world was ending this evening against a celestial clock waiting for another sun to rise.

When the *John Harvey* combusted, it took Lieutenant Richardson, Lieutenant Beckstrom, and his six chemical warfare men—and the remainder of the crew on duty. Snap of a whip, and they were gone.

At this moment, no one was aware that the cunning and nearly invisible mustard gas was stealthily applying more havoc than was apparent. The monster you can't see in a horror movie but you know is lurking. Steadfast. Relentless. Pervasive. Grinning! Drooling through Bari's streets, and edifices. The screams, moans, and bleating, the pleas for help, the incessant soundtrack with no pending, thunderous finale: *Tosca, Act III. Tannhäuser: Overture.*

Forty-foot-high flames with thick black smoke covered the East Jetty, making it almost impossible to breathe. And it would spread throughout the harbor. Many ships motionless, waiting at the bloodied chopping block for another German bomb to explode.

And so, the Ju 88s had been into the mission for just ten minutes; they would circle back, sharks coming round again for a second and third taste and continue bombing and strafing for the next ten minutes.

An eternity.

The Germans, all of them flying that day, including the non-flying strategic planners Peltz and von Richthofen, had no notion of the full scope their bombing mission would have on Bari on 2 December 1943—on the world, on history. They set out to bomb a harbor filled with Allied ships stuffed with war equipment to dislodge the German grip on the Italian peninsula and end a war that the Germans were tenaciously perpetuating despite their dwindling assets and prospects.

Their mission was simple, essentially: Bomb the merchant ships in Bari's harbor. And so, when they came back to their airfields in their intact bombers and bloodless flying suits and cheered and celebrated with German gusto, they felt justified in hailing themselves for a mission well-accomplished. They rendered terrific havoc on the ships and certainly curtailed the distribution of necessary supplies, temporarily, for the Allie's war effort. Their forces, too, went haphazardly beyond the harbor's perimeter and extended into the city of Bari. There was not a pane of glass in the immediate vicinity left unshattered. The streets were a snow of glass.

But none of the German crews or generals, at that moment of celebratory joy, knew of the unintentional side effect of their bombing—knew the effective spread of the vaporous secret, the garlic, the escape of the horror far more pervasive and damaging than bombs and bullets.

The only people who knew with certainty were the dead and dying.

What is the law on gas weapons?

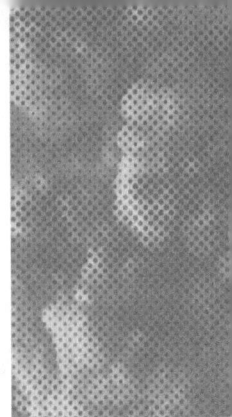

10

THE DEVIL'S DOING

The harbor a grim mien.

At the breakwater, bodies swirled in the tide. A ship's wake swirled the water, and disfigured bodies lolled. The surface of the harbor was a foot of oil, indiscernible debris and dunnage with varying sizes of oil fires flickering on the surface. Bodies floating on the scum showed yellow skin coloring. The harbor and the city presented a tableau of devastation and hell that could have only been invoked by Hades, the god of the dead himself. From many perspectives, the harbor and destroyed, skeletal ships appeared to replicate the Japanese attack at Pearl Harbor in December 1941. The two attacks comparable: surprise attacks, overwhelming forces of enemy aircraft at an innocuous hour of the day, and a number of excessive deaths and injuries that strangled medical and emergency facilities. The chaos was so similar that the attack at Bari would quickly and forever become known as the "Little Pearl Harbor."

In a letter to Gerald Reminick, author of *Nighmare in Bari* (see Bibliography), George Maury, the assistant engineer of the SS *Lyman Abbott*, stated:

When all the fury of the explosion subsided, there was a deathly silence except for moans and cries of the wounded and dying. A lot of blood was coming from my nose and ears [from the concussive force of the explosions], which also blew my shoes off my feet.

One piece of shrapnel entered my mouth, went through my upper jaw, fractured it, and came out under my left eye. I had intense pain in my lower left rib and found that I couldn't put weight on my left leg. The Coxswain gave orders to abandon the ship.

I looked out at the harbor, which was on fire, and survival did not seem possible to me> When we headed for shore in the lifeboat, ships were exploding, bombs were still screaming down, and there was fire everywhere. One of the ships was riding high in the water and coming right at us. We managed to get around it, and I will never know how we got to shore.

I found myself on the ground above the shoreline, trying to figure out what that strange smell was [garlic]. Two British soldiers picked me up and carried me to a Jeep. One of them looked at me and said, "We had a bit of a bloody time, didn't we, sailor?" I didn't answer...

And here, also a piece of Reminick's research, a partial Anti-Aircraft Action Summary report filed by Capt. Hays of the *Aroostock*:

The sky was lit up bright, even, then day, and the Commanding Officer could clearly see the effort being exerted on his ship against the enemy. What appeared to be the most effective and most consistent barrage of any activity in the harbor area was maintained by the U.S.S. *Aroostock* until firing ceased. The sky was filled with flying sparks, burning debris, with much shrapnel and other missiles being hurtled through the air and falling white-hot, into the water, on the ships, and on the quay. At least three bombs were seen to explode in the water close astern the U.S.S. *Aroostock* throwing larger geysers of watch into the air and onto the ship.

Two ships, [Polish registered *Lwow* and *Puck* anchored within 260 yards and 400 yards, respectively, of the *Aroostock* sustained direct hits and immediately sank in about (4 ½) to (6) fathoms of water, the upper decks and superstructure still burning fiercely …

Approximately two hours after the action started, a large ammunition ship exploded with 375 yards of the U.S.S. *Aroostook*, the impact of the explosion causing considerable superficial damages to the ship, and momentarily stunning everyone in exposed position. The Commanding Officer, about 700 yards distant from the exploding ship, was nearly blown into the sea from the quay and suffered partial deafness.

The next morning, 3 December, the British Port Commandant, the leading military authority in Bari, informed higher command that there was a risk of mustard gas in the harbor. Because of this, he recommended that the *John Harvey* be immediately scuttled. This was a moot point because, obviously, the commandant had not seen the *Harvey* in the harbor; actually, there was not much *Harvey* to see. For the most part, the ship no longer existed. After her explosion, her mustard gas had spread with stealth and rapidity through the air, the water; an undetermined number of shattered mustard shells sank. Her charred and twisted masts and upper structure were the only signs that the ship was anything but an apparition.

The commandant's word spread quickly to the 98th General Hospital regarding the possibility of mustard gas in the harbor. In turn, the detail was spread to the hospital's causality stations: "The PAD Officer No. 6 Base Sub area visited the docks and reported to his HQ at about 0900 hrs. that mustard gas had been smelled in the dock area. About 0930 hrs., HQ No. 2 District telephoned and confirmed some gas was in the dock area." One hour later, the British Base Military Officer stated, "the first definite knowledge he had about gas was on 3 Dec. about 1030 hrs. He went around with the Port Defense Officer to the site suspected of contamination. He boarded the HMS *Vienna*, where he found that sickbay personnel had their eyes affected and the doctor, a blister on one foot."

Now begins controversy, secrecy, misinformation, and the devil's doing, duplicity.

Here, it is important to note that the presence of conflicting information abounds. Around midnight, casualties began arriving at hospitals from the harbor area:

The hospitals [note plural] were puzzled by the nature of some of the casualties they were receiving and their subsequent development. Such warning as they may have received about the possible presence of gas certainly did not reach the appropriate quarters, and there is some evidence that, on a telephone inquiry being made by 98 Gen. Hospital (where the majority of casualties were) to Navy House on the morning of 3 Dec., *no confirmation of the presence of mustard* [emphasis added] gas in the harbor could be obtain. Whether the alleged informant was ignorant of the facts or was *impressed with a supposed desirability of secrecy is not clear* [emphasis added].

Throughout the night and early morning, ambulance sirens ululated incessantly, transporting afflicted Allied personnel to hospitals. For the most part, Bari's citizens were ignored by the British and Americans; they had to tend to themselves. First came medical care for military personnel, US Navy Army, and so forth.

Bombs that willy-nilly missed the harbor hit the old part of the city's buildings, leaving them damaged. In *A History of the Twenty-Sixth General Hospital,* "Shattered glass littered the streets. Steel shutters covering shop windows were twisted and ripped off. The roofs and sides of buildings were caved in. Huge fragments of metal lay in the streets. It was no wonder that the civilian population were terrified!" A mass exit ensued, and terror spread throughout the populace. "Woman carried bundles on their heads. Some refugees led a goat or sheep on a leash. Everyone was frightened. Where they were going, we do not know, but they were intent on leaving the city behind. No one seemed to know how many civilians were killed during the raid, but the number of casualties must have been high."

The *Chicago Daily News* was the first to print a descriptive account; the secret had started to collapse:

Long before daylight the harried civilian population took to the roads in a panic resembling that of the last day of France. By noon little boys and girls on bicycles or scooter or afoot were slowly moving toward their aunts and uncles and other relatives who lived in greater security along the interior highways

High-wheeled carts from the olive groves had been pressed into service and Bari's people in steadily increasing numbers, had started one of those treks that never get anywhere. It was like hiking the retreat to Bordeaux all over again to watch them—serious-faced oldsters and clusters of little children, all mounted high on cartloads of pitiful household trash, sewing machines, post and pans, chairs, tables, pitchforks, shovels and bedding—always sewing machines and bedding.

On the docks that morning about 25 badly burned British and American sailors sat outside the navy house waiting for someone to take them somewhere else, They had been unable to get into any of the overcrowded hospitals and had been treated right where they were. They were foul with refuse of the harbor and streaked with the horrible purple dyes of burn unguents ...

Immediate treatment in all the overcrowded hospitals was rudimentary at best. In too many cases, there was no time to formally admit a patient, interview them, or bed them with a hospital gown. Oily wet clothing remained clinging to them. Immediate treatment was to wrap them in a blanket for twenty-four hours and give them a hot cup of tea; they were not washed or cleaned. There was insufficient time and too many casualties to tend to. By the second day, more than 800 Allied casualties were hospitalized. More than 650 had mustard burns.

On the first night, many of the cases were not admitted to a hospital. They appeared in good condition and so were sent to an Auxiliary Seaman's Home still in their soiled clothing, the mustard gas soaked clothing clinging to their skin. The next morning, they were finally admitted to hospitals—then the symptoms of mustard gas poisoning started to develop with a vengeance.

Sending these patients to an auxiliary home and still clad in their soiled clothes was not medical personnel's fault, not an oversight. At this point, no signs of mustard gas poisoning appeared. And even if it did, medical personnel, technicians, and doctors had no idea nor any experience in mustard gas poisoning or how to treat the symptoms.

Leaving the uniforms on the patients only hastened the absorption rate of mustard into the body. This oversight was exactly the opposite treatment for a mustard gas victim.

In the "Medical Report of the Bari Harbor Mustard Gas Causalities" published in *The Military Surgeon*, Lt. Col. Stewart F. Alexander wrote, "The first indication of an unusual type of causality that evening was noted in the resuscitation wards. Casualties that supposedly were suffering from shock following immersion and exposure did not appear to fit the usual clinical picture and did not respond to plasma, pain-killing drugs, and were generally apathetic."

But six hours after the attack, the horrors began escalating when patients started having complications in their eyes. Some became practically blinded tearful, almost all saying that the pain was more severe than having sand in them.

The burns evolved into hideous blisters and appeared in patients who had been in contact with the harbor water. Their genital areas were obviously more vulnerable from floating in the harbor and swelled many times their normal proportions and were deeply painful.

And what about the citizens of Bari?

They were the last in line for any treatment. All the resources were in the hands of the British and American forces—hospitals, doctors, ambulances, medical supplies. And intentions to take care of their own came first.

While no records were kept of casualties, an estimate puts the deaths at more than 1,000 to 2,000 military and civilians killed in the attack—from the mustard gas and the results of bombing and strafing. It will never be known how many Barites went untreated for mustard gas inhalation and burns or complications. Nor how many were killed resulting from the bombs dropped haphazardly. As stated, it was not the German's intent to bomb the city; they wanted to save their sparse bombs and bullets for the ships in the harbor, which posed a direct threat to them. Bari, the city, had no military value; it would have been folly to bomb the streets and buildings in the city when the merchant ships had cargo that could have been used against them in combat.

During this initial period, military casualties were diagnosed as "Dermartis NYD," showing the blisters on the skin were "Not Yet Diagnosed."

Soon, a suspicion questioned the symptoms—chemical warfare was becoming the dominant suspect. Of course, the blame was placed on the Germans and their raid that evening.

Naturally, the paramount question arose: What type of chemical was it? Further, Did the Germans drop mustard gas on ships *and* the city? Or did the Allies have mustard gas cargos aboard their ships that they were keeping secret? These were questions a garden variety detective would have asked—questions of importance whose answers could have helped in the proper treatment.

* * *

The sun rose mordantly on Bari on 4 December, and it was generally agreed that the situation needed the immediate intervention of a higher, medically superior authority that those available at Bari, an expert in chemical warfare—the situation was beyond the normal capabilities of the medical personnel at the city. Naturally, many of the patients started to panic, feeling that they were going permanently blind or their genitals were being destroyed.

A call for help rang out.

Deputy Chief Surgeon General Fred Blesse of the Allied Headquarters in Algiers dispatched Lt. Col. Steward F. Alexander, who would be the crucial force in recognizing and spearheading the mustard gas problem. But Blesse first had to contact Gen. Eisenhower for permission to dispatch Alexander, and only after Eisenhower had him swear to take a military oath to keep the incident secret—which seemed natural but risky. How could they keep hundreds of patients, doctors, and naval personnel from speaking about the possibilities of mustard gas?

Alexander flew to Bari and began an immediate tour of the hospitals.

Born and raised in Park Ridge, New Jersey on 30 Aug. 1914 (not far from where this narrative was written), Col. Stewart Francis Alexander was a medical doctor and expert in chemical warfare. After graduating from Staunton Military Academy and Dartmouth College, he received his medical degree in 1937 from Columbia University in New York City.

He had worked on mustard gas warfare at the Edgewood Arsenal in Maryland and quickly surmised what the culprit in

Bari was. At the same time, he knew the shipment to Bari was top secret. Now, he had been placed in a difficult position: reveal the secret and help the patients and encourage the Germans to deliver a counterattack of mustard gas or keep the secret to the detriment of the patients?

Almost instantly, Lt. Col. Alexander's astute nostrils gave him the first piece of solid evidence as to what had occurred at the harbor.

The smell of mustard gas.

Working with measured haste, he viewed chest X-rays, blisters, and sputum. He soon recognized that the problem was definitely caused by mustard gas. However, he could not pinpoint if it was liquid or vaporized mustard, nor the method of delivery, because the harbor water had diluted most of the evidence.

These were important points in his investigation because they would have quickly led to the source and, thus, the approach to mitigate the problem. Press on he did.

And doing so with dogged energy, the so-called "mustard gas incident" began evolving into one of the disasters of WWII, albeit one of its least known even to this day.

Winston Churchill's position on the gas incident was to keep the presence of mustard gas secret, despite the fact that Blesse had informed him of the incident, both to prevent public outcry and to avoid potentially provoking the Germans into retaliatory chemical attacks. Churchill, along with other Allied leaders, feared that admitting the presence of mustard gas could escalate the use of chemical weapons in the war, which all sides had largely refrained from using due to the Geneva Protocol and the potential for mutual destruction.

Churchill, Eisenhower, and the Allied leaders quickly agreed to keep the mustard gas aspect of the Bari disaster classified. Public knowledge of the incident could have led to intense criticism and a backlash, as well as concerns from both the military and the public regarding the Allies' readiness to use chemical weapons.

Churchill was particularly concerned that Germany, if aware of Allied chemical stockpiling in Italy, might view it as a green light to deploy chemical weapons against Allied forces or civilians in retaliation. Maintaining secrecy was a strategic decision aimed at containing the situation and avoiding using chemicals to fight the war.

And so, official denial crept into the scenario: Allied commanders, under the directive to keep this information secret, issued public statements "attributing the casualties solely to the bombing and avoided any mention of chemical exposure."

Churchill supported this narrative to prevent the spread of panic or political fallout.

At the same time, medical secrecy and limited treatment resources—initially, medical personnel—were not informed of the mustard gas exposure, which resulted in delayed and inadequate treatment for those affected. As a result, many more died from a lack of honesty and proper attention.

Within two weeks of the bombing, *The Washington Post* broke the story, not only of the attack but the devastating causality rate. They called it the costliest "sneak attack" since Pearl Habor:

Secretary of War Simpson had intended to release a few details at his weekly press conference. But after the *Post* story, newsmen found him sizzling. His anger seemed greater than was justified by a mere premature news "leak." He was brusque, stiff, and cut the conference short. When a reporters wanted to know if the Allies had actually been caught napping [they were], Stimson replied: "No! I will not comment on this thing."

The news from Bari was bad. What was even worse was the skittishness in Washington (or London) about telling the facts. If, after four years of World War II, the people of the U.S. should come finally to believe that their leaders are unwilling to trust them to "take" bad news, that disaster would be greater than any Bari.

The Germans, of course, saw the incident as a windfall and jumped on it immediately for propaganda purposes—but, thankfully, held off in retaliating. Prior to the bombing run, they had no idea what they were going to cause that evening. By sheer chance, their bombing attack on the ships was responsible for releasing the poison gas. However, there is no record of regret on their part. They were able to use the release of the gas to gain a psychological advantage. Subsequent to the Bari bombing, Axis Sally, broadcasting from Berlin, sarcastically said, "I see you boys are getting gassed up by your own poison gas."

Axis Sally, actually Mildred Gillars, a German American, was the generic nickname given to two female radio personalities who broadcast English-language propaganda on behalf of the European Axis Powers during World War II—both used the pseudonym Axis Sally. Gillars was the first woman in U.S. history to be convicted of treason by the United States following her arrest in Berlin on 8 March 1949; she was sentenced to ten to thirty years imprisonment. She would alternate between broadcasting swing music and propaganda aimed at American troops. Her main message was surrender, your girlfriends are home cheating on you, and the Axis powers know all your locations. American soldiers listened to Gillar's broadcasts for popular music but found her propaganda efforts a joke.

Not much of the world seemed to be yearning to get a picture of what happened at Bari on 2 December. Apparently, because of the desire for secrecy, there was not an overwhelming news of what occurred. However, on 16 December, *The New York Times* published the most up-to-date report:

NAZIS SANK 17 SHIPS IN BOMBING OF BARI

Capital Hears Still Others Were Hit—
Stimson Shields Data—Casualties 1,000

By Sydney Shalett
Special to The New York Times

WASHINGTON, Dec 16—The successful German air attack on the Italian port of Bari at dawn on Dec. 2 was revealed today by Secretary of War Henry Stimson as a disaster of considerable magnitude in which a "number" of Allied vessels, including two ammunition ships and five American merchantmen [a ship used in commerce] were destroyed or damaged and 1,000 casualties occurred.

Mr. Stimson, obviously angry over certain circumstance preceding his announcement, including a premature "breaking" of the story by The Washington Post, gave only a sketchy account of the happenings at Bari, and irately refused to give any further details.

Informed sources in the capital indicated, however, that the Allied losses were even greater than those revealed by the War Department. It was stated that seventeen Allied ships were lost, exclusive of others that may have been damaged.

Bari, some 125 miles behind the front lines on the Adriatic coast, lies on a portion of the Italian peninsula were Gen. Sir Bernard L. Montgomery's Eighth Army, fighting under Gen. Dwight D. Eisenhower's overall command, is dominant. There was reason to believe that the Germans might have caught Allied defenses there off guard.

[The Associated Press suggested the German force comprised about thirty plans.]

Mr. Stimson, taking up the story in the course of a war review that he reads to correspondents at his weekly press conference, prefaces his account by explaining that, while we have "definite air superiority throughout southern Italy and over most of the Mediterranean," the Germans have "appreciably increased their air strength in this area." Some "heavy German bomber raids" on our shipping and port facilities have occurred," he observed.

Munitions Ships Explode

"In the German air raid of Dec. 2, on the southern Italian port of Bari, Allied shipping in the harbor was heavily damaged," Mr. Stimson related. "Two ammunition ships were hit and the resultant explosions caused spreading fires which destroyed or damaged a number of Allied cargo ships and small harbor craft.

"Among the vessels destroyed were five American merchantmen. Fortunately, most of the cargoes had been discharged prior to the attack. Consequently, the loss of supplies was not great. There were an estimated 1,000 casualties, including thirty-seven American naval personnel. This raid was originally announced by General Eisenhower in his communiqué of Dec.4."

[The Associated Pess said that there were about thirty Allied ships in the harbor at the time of the attack.]

The communiqué to which Mr. Stimson referred, after dealing with accounts of various actions by American forces, stated at the end: "On the evening of Dec. 2 enemy aircraft attacked the Bari area and damage was done. There were a number of casualties."

It is reliably reported in the capital that the Office of War Information had favored putting out a more detailed account of the Bari incident, partly on he theory that, within the limits of security, news of disasters as well as victories should be given to the American public, and partly because the OWI thought that we should get out news first from our sources and not from the enemy.

Mr. Stimson declined to identify the nationality of the ammunition ships that started the holocaust; declined to give any further information about ship losses other than what he read and declined to state whether the thirty-seven naval personnel were all Americans killed. He said concerning this last point that the War Department does not have full information on the casualties.

Finally, when a reporter started to ask him if he would comment on reports that Bari defenders had been caught off guard, Mr. Stimson cut him off before he could finish his question.

"No! I will not comment on this thing!"

It is highly likely that Stimson was in the loop regarding the secrecy attached to the mustard gas. During the press conference it appears he was worried about the mustard would pop up. He did not. Nevertheless, he shut down the conference merely by saying he was not going to comment further. And that was about as far as any revelation about mustard gas got out to the public.

On April 8, 1944, four months after the Bari attack, the *Army and Navy Register* printed a letter to the managing editor of the *Kansas City Star* and president of the American Society of Newspaper Editors concerning the U.S. Army's news policy. In the letter, Major General A.D. Surles, the U.S. Army Director of Public Relations, stated the public's sentiment:

"I can sense the growing idea that we are endeavoring to cover up mistakes and either in the guise of military security, and yet it is difficult to counteract this impression in view of the fact that the problem complicated the need for the theater commandeer to use information as a psychological weapon against the enemy, and because of the necessity for the theater commander to maintain high morale among troops whom are in physical contact with the enemy, I must confess that we, here at home, are in poor position to judge national interest in terms of these ramifications…"

Notable is the fact that the British had overall command of Bari—they unequivocally knew that the *Harvey* had sailed into the harbor with mustard gas. A significant point because, publicly, the British consistently denied any knowledge of the *Harvey's* pernicious cargo, following the lead proffered by Winston Churchill, who vehemently denied that mustard gas was present in Bari.

The Americans, on the other hand, were more pragmatically inclined and thought reasonably so that they could not keep the poison a secret and that sooner or later, the facts would dribble out. And dribble they did.

Part of the "strategy of containment," obviously dubious, involved ships leaving the harbor: they departed carrying news that the fires were started by anything other than mustard gas and it was the fires that "burned" the victims' skin. Not surprisingly, the news spread rapidly to Augusta, Brindisi, and Taranto. Thus, a complex situation now created acts of deliberate disinformation that only further confused the chaos and suffering at Bari.

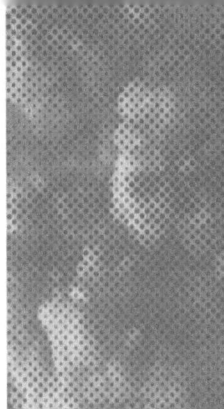

11

BURNS—"NOT YET DETERMINED"

After spending the day making hospital rounds and carefully examining dozens of gas victims, Col. Alexander was practically convinced that the affected were suffering from mustard poisoning. Years as a medical doctor and working in chemical warfare supported his thesis. But he needed more proof to sell it to the higher-ups—and even then, he knew it would be difficult to convince them. The authorities were adamant about toeing the line, keeping the mustard gas effect a secret—and there were careers at stake. Further, Alexander felt that if he pushed too hard, his efforts could lead to a court-martial or a transfer. This was insinuated more than once.

Initially, he divided his conclusions into two groupings: those with severe external chemical burns and those with internal damage caused by ingestion or inhalation of mustard, harbor water, or both. Also, the situation was exacerbated when the victims were pulled from the harbor, wrapped in blankets, and continuously inhaled mustard vapors soaked in the blanket.

The more he learned, the more Alexander understood how the mustard became so profuse.

First, he concluded—and most important—that "a German airborne delivery was most unlikely."

Second, politically speaking, he was one hundred percent sure that the Germans would not, at this stage of the war, weaponize mustard poison—particularly after their horrendous experiences they experienced during WWI.

He reviewed the other methods in which mustard could be used, hoping that if any of the equipment or weapons used in dispersing the agent were on a ship's manifest in the harbor on 2 Dec., he could nail down the epicenter. He was more than familiar with ground delivery methods, familiar with the Army's 4.2-inch mortar shell that contained mustard.

He would not accept how the Ju 88s could have dropped enough gas bombs or use spray tanks to inflict the kinds of injuries he was seeing; the injuries, highly pervasive, covered the entire harbor and invaded the city. This meant civilians were suffering, too. Soon, he concluded that an aerial delivery by the Germans was out of the question.

He moved on.

While he was doing his investigative work, he figured it was imperative to get autopsies on the men who had already died from "burns n.y.d"—burns "not yet determined."

Next, he undertook an extremely tedious task: Using a drawing pad and pencil, he began outling a diagram of Bari's harbor as precisely as he could, sketching each ship's position on the night of 2 Dec. The port's authorities provided the necessary details to complete his sketch (harbors layout, dimensions, etc), marking each ship's location. He was certain that if such a chart showed a preponderance of deaths in one location, then the ship in that location should be investigated as a prime carrier of the toxic gas. Then, he would the ship's cago manifest to determine if mustard was aboard.

Meanwhile, many people were dying, and a few authorities would speak to him when the subject came up. Alexander was justifiably furious.

He then carefully started to question the British authorities, also all reluctant to answer him. "Everyone," he later wrote, "including the Post Commander, denied the presence of American or British mustard gas."

Essentially, the Allies were doing what they had been trained to do throughout their careers: obey orders and keep silent at all costs, even if it involved the lives of their colleagues and the citizens of Bari. This was almost standard operating procedure for any military.

Then, fate intervened.

A diver searching the harbor floor found multiple fractured shells resembling gas bombs. Tests taken immediately on site revealed traces of mustard. American ordnance officers from Doolittle's Fifteenth Air Force were immediately pulled in and identified a casing from a 100-pound American M47A2 mustard gas bomb. It was immediately evident that the Germans did not manufacture this casing: German mustard gas bombs were always marked with a distinctive *Gelb Kreuz* (yellow cross indicating mustard gas).

Alexander's instincts were right: he concluded that an Allied merchant ship—the *John Harvey*—had been carrying a large cargo of mustard gas. He rightfully deduced that the bombs were destined for a secret chemical stockpile at nearby Foggia, the new home of Doolittle's Fifteenth Air Force, where, if necessary, they could have been loaded into B-17 and B-24 bombers and dropped wherever and whenever if necessary.

Alexander's training at Edgewood told him the M47 was a simple sheet-metal bomb (1/32nd of an inch thick), about four feet long and eight inches in diameter, primarily designed to hold white phosphorus or liquid sulfur mustard. It went into military use in the 1930s along with many problems, including the thin sheet-metal casing, which was easily ruptured and prone to leakage. Alexander knew that the traditional German bombs dropped from the Ju 88s would have blown the gas bombs to pieces during the attack, releasing the lethal mustard into the harbor and the atmosphere around the city.

He was getting closer to solving the mysteries that prevailed.

But there was a speed bump: Alexander's discovery that the mustard gas emanated from the "Allies own supply" was now making his job more difficult, more political.

The 29-year-old doctor now found himself in the middle of a diplomatic crisis, a situation he was embroiled in from the moment he arrived a couple of days ago. And the matter also had a "frightful international import."

There was no question that this situation was a "self-inflicted wound" caused by the Allies. Attempts by the British to obfuscate and possibly conceal evidence vexed, yes, but that was minor compared to their effort to shift responsibility for the spread of mustard gas to the Luftwaffe. He winced to think that "If they [the Allies] were going to accuse the Germans of dropping mustard when the Germans had not...there would be grave political implications."

His anxiety ascended.

Then, on Friday, 10 December, mustard gas deaths suddenly spiked. That evening, by the time Alexander left the hospital, nine men had died in a twenty-four-hour period. This was difficult and incomprehensible for the hospital staff to accept—even though Alexander had correctly diagnosed the toxic agent and arranged for the proper treatment.

Alexander felt an urgent need now to inform AFHQ, Gen. Beeles, in Algiers and give him an executive view of his initial findings. He wrote his memo nine days after the bombing; it was brief and to the point:

T.C.C 1215 hrs.

The burns in the hospitals in this area labeled "dermatitis n.y.d." are due to mustard gas. They are unusual types and varieties because most of them are due to mustard which has been mixed into the surface oil in the harbor.

There are three factors to be considered in appraising the deaths that have occurred in the group:

1. Blast injury
2. Immersion and exposure
3. Mustard poisoning

In the majority of the cases I believe the mustard poisoning is the most important factor.

There are still many cases seriously ill, some of whom I am sure will die.

>(sgd.) STEWART F. ALEXANDER
>Lt. Colonel, M.C.,
>Consultant
>11 DEC 43.

By the end of that day, nineteen more men had perished.

Now, Alexander saw it suitable to take an unprecedented action for a lieutenant colonel—he would appeal directly to the President of the United States, Franklin Roosevelt, and Prime Minster Churchill, a highly unorthodox move. Because he had met Roosevelt and Churchill in person at the Casablanca Conference, he felt this extraordinary action was the best course to take. He expected no response but was surprised when Roosevelt responded: "Please keep me fully informed."

But Churchill was not impressed with Alexander's "medical detective snooping"—or, at least he would not admit to Alexander's findings. Later, he would admit that that he felt the doctor was "snooping around" in an area best left to higher authorities. Reacting, Churchill sent a memo out stating, "your man in the field must have made a mistake" and that he, Churchill, did not believe there was mustard gas in Bari. He asked that the situation be reevaluated.

Alexander was gobsmacked.

Because Churchill decided to keep the gas detail top secret, he instead attributed all the deaths to "burns due to enemy action"—such as shrapnel, fire, bullets, and explosions. This decision by the British and the Americans made an exact count of the deaths impossible. Further, revealing the details to General Eisenhower also added to the number of deaths because Eisenhower took no action to treat for mustard gas. Generally, if the medical personnel did not know what the patients were dying from, no treatment could be efficaciously applied.

Can we blame Churchill?

Can we blame Eisenhower?

Their action, or lack of it, to support secrecy certainly led to an increase in deaths. However, it also prevented the initiation of mustard gas warfare on both sides—Allies and Axis.

Despite the fact that he had proof, conclusive proof, Alexander saw no point in arguing with the messenger. Colonels don't argue with presidents or prime ministers.

Certainly, British medical personnel in Bari were not going to follow Alexander's lead unless it was approved in London at Downing Street. All were in a quandary. What to do?

Col. Alexander was losing sleep over this question—and others.

Churchill, ever astute, pointed to the most important questions about the Bari victims: Why were the effects in this group of mustard casualties more profound than any other recorded in military history? Why were they unrecognized by the Allied doctors and by Churchill?

Alexander's calculations showed that more patients were dying at Bari than had on the battlefields of World War I, where the fatality rate had been approximately two percent among those hospitalized with gas injuries. However, in Bari, that number was many times higher—close to 13 percent of the casualties proving fatal—and before it all ended, it would rise even higher.

Why?

The reason: Because the dispersal of mustard gas at Bari was different (direct contact) than that suffered by British troops at Ypres (asphyxia). At Bari, few people suffered from gas inhalation alone, so the massive pulmonary congestion characteristics of victims of World War I were only "minimally present."

What was different about the Bari victims was the amount of mustard absorbed through the skin from lengthy, intimate contact from immersion in the oily harbor water, their clothing, and the blankets they were wrapped in.

After the *Harvey* exploded, many of the seamen aboard either jumped or were blown off into the oily mustard gas water along with people who were dockside. This caused a massive number of casualties—both via the mustard gas as well as impact from shrapnel.

Alexander hypothesized: "The individuals, to all intents and purposes, were dipped into a solution of mustard-in-oil, and then wrapped in blankets, given warm tea, and allowed a long period for absorption. Never before had any doctor or medical researcher encountered such an extraordinary level of mustard gas toxicity." These were optimal conditions that permitted such "significant exposures," and that led to this unique form of poisoning.

* * *

There was no bright side to the misery and deaths at Bari, one of the worst naval disasters of the war after Pearl Harbor. Compounding this was that much of the truth surrounding the attack and the mustard gas involvement was being deliberately suppressed from the world and, more important, from Col. Alexander, who was there to care for the wounded and dying.

The news of Bari, *Time* magazine wrote, "was the skittishness in Washington (or London) about telling the facts."

It was starting to become apparent that whatever happened at Bari was no ordinary event in the war so far and that there was a concerted effort to suppress the nature of what really occurred.

Essentially, there were two attacks on 2 Dec.: the Luftwaffe and their bombers, bombs, and strafing, and the secondary explosion of the mustard gas bombs coming from the SS *John Harvey*. One seemed to be worse than the other.

Further, on a larger, more significant scale, the destruction and ruination at Bari prolonged the war, precluded the delivery of vital supplies, and hobbled Doolittle's Fifteenth Air Force in Foggia. It would take many weeks to replenish all the lost supplies that were destroyed in the attack—this included the pending landings at Normandy, France, several months away in June of 1944. Supplies coming through Bari that had been destined for the Normandy invasion had to be reordered, which took more time.

And, of course, there was the gossip mill and numerous conspiracy theories attributed to the Germans, the Americans, and the British.

Rumors blossomed as they would when facts were stifled. There was speculation that censorship abounded and that the War Department was holding back the actual losses because they did not want to diminish morale across the nation—or indicate to the Germans that a US merchant ship containing 2,000 tons of mustard gas bombs was docked in Bari.

There was speculation, too, that the Germans had utilized a new, rocket-driven glide bomb with spectacular results.

Robert Casey, a reporter for the United Press, wrote that "One glance at the line of merchant ships and one had to know that the port would be 'marked with a large red tack on the Germans operation map.'"

And the pool reporters would never let go of Coningham's outlandish, uncorroborated boast on the morning of the attack during his press conference. Even the U.S. Navy was blamed (perhaps rightfully so) for allowing so many "valuable eggs in one small basket for such a dividend of destruction, particularly when enemy bases were just across the narrow Adriatic."

In the middle of it all, even General Eisenhower got caught up in the matter and asked a special Senate committee to investigate the horrible setback in lives and equipment—despite the fact that he certainly knew that the SS *John Harvey* was loaded with 2,000 tons of mustard gas bombs.

Particularly aggrieved was Rear Admiral Emory Scott Land, the war shipping administrator responsible for the US merchant marine fleet across seven seas. He told *Time* magazine: "You're going to hear more about that raid before you hear less." Of course, his was not the last word, and the matter continued to skip along, shrouded in mystery and duplicity.

Meanwhile, almost all the participants—the victims, hospital technicians, politicians, naval personnel, etc.—never dreamed that it would be almost thirty years before they heard the truth. Wartime secrecy made the matter much worse than it was; it always does.

But it was that wartime secrecy of the Bari incident and the determined efforts of American and British governments to cover up the incident so as to not endanger the preparation of the most important operation of the war, Overlord, the Allied invasion of German-occupied France planned for June 1944.

Certainly, it was a lesson in underestimating the enemy.

Col. Alexander, by this time, had nearly completed his "Final Report of the Bari Mustard Gas Causalities" findings, which was released on 20 June 1944. While extremely lengthy and highly technical, there are significant passages that serve this narrative. Particularly paragraph 3 in which the colonel indirectly "blames" Prime Minister Winston Churchill for keeping the matter untouchable. He wrote:

It is most necessary to point out that none of the medical case sheets make any mention of a vesicant [blister] agent because of the security regulations applied [by Churchill] at the time. The use of the term "N.Y.D. [Not Yet Determined] Dermatitis" was a command decision [imposed by Churchill]. It is to be regretted that the tremendous pressure under which the hospitals were working prevented the accomplishments that were desired and requested at the time. By the same virtue, certain of the recorded case sheets are scanty in relation to the observations that were actually made.

Wise it was for Col. Alexander to keep Churchill's name

cloaked and office from the report, thus certainly saving his neck from further humiliation, censure, and possible insubordination.

At this point Alexander felt the issue of mysterious deaths at Bari had been solved.

One item that convinced him that he was correct was his detailed sketch of the harbor that he had made with the cooperation of the British authorities, the US military, dockworkers, and anyone who had an association with the project. By identifying and questioning the victims, the sketch indicated the location of the ship that contained the mustard gas that evening and what ship they were aboard—the SS *John Harvey*. Simultaneously, when the *Harvey* exploded, it killed dozens of people—civilian and military—who had been on the dock adjacent to the ship. Thus, Alexander's detailed sketch showed that the greatest number of mustard-induced deaths occurred among the people closest to the ship—the *Harvey*— (designated Ship 1 on Alexander's detailed map), and those on adjacent ships.

The report was widely distributed throughout the medical community throughout the United States medically community, such that it is considered even today a landmark in the history of mustard poisoning. Now that Alexander knew what the toxic agent was, that it was aboard the SS *John Harvey*, an American ship, he felt that his assignment in Bari was satisfactorily accomplished. He could return to his headquarters at the Office of the Surgeon, Headquarters, North African Theatre of Operations, Algiers. Once there, he began issuing reports about the medical aspects of his findings. At the same time, he began sending out his findings, advising authorities that they should be prepared for any future incidents. Once again, one of the respondents to the reports was Winston Churchill, whose reply was instantaneous, persistent, and staunch: "The symptoms do not sound like mustard gas." This reaction was the second time Alexander received a similar response from Churchill.

Then, for the sake of cooperation between the British and Americans, British officials suggested that "the cause of the chemical burns should just be labeled 'NYD–Not Yet Diagnosed." All the medical officers, including Alexander, refused to change the report, replying that their professional integrity was at stake

More important, after a detailed study of tissue blocks at the Edgewood Arsenal in Maryland, they were sent to scientists at Yale University, "noting that there was no doubt that the mustard had damaged the lymphatic system and the bone marrow of the victims. These observations immediately suggest *the significance of compounds of this type for the possible treatment of neoplastic* [abnormal growth] *disorders of the tissue that form white blood cells* [emphasis added]."

The mustard gases were tested at Yale as bone marrow depressants in the treatment of certain human tumors. Also, Hodgkins's disease and leukemia were good possible candidates for the application of the powerful agent.

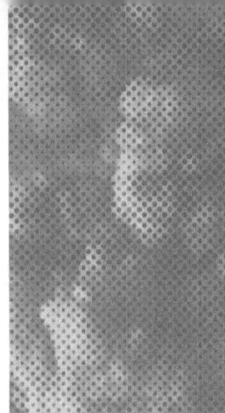

12

THE FATHER OF CHEMOTHERAPY

To this day, there is no current drug or treatment that cures all forms of cancer.

The effect of most drugs and other cancer actions effect restores a degree of health and prolongs life—the experimenting, however, continues.

As of this writing, January 2025, The American Cancer Society has released its annual Cancer Statistics report for the year, highlighting notable trends in cancer incidence and mortality. While the overall cancer death rate in the U.S. has decreased by 34 percent since 1991—translating to approximately 4.5 million fewer deaths—there are concerning increases in cancer incidence among certain demographics.

Rising Cancer Rates in Women: Historically, men had higher cancer rates, primarily due to higher smoking prevalence.

However, recent data indicate that women, especially those under 65, are now more likely than men to develop cancer. This shift is attributed to increases in breast and lung cancer cases among women.

Increased Incidence in Younger Populations: Women under 50 now face an 82 percent higher cancer incidence rate compared to their male counterparts, up from 51 percenet higher in 2002. This rise is largely driven by breast and thyroid cancers.

Lung Cancer Trends: For the first time, lung cancer incidence among women under 65 has surpassed that of men. This is partly because women began smoking heavily later than men and have been slower to quit, leading to a delayed decline in lung cancer rates among women.

Contributing Factors: The increase in cancer cases among women and younger populations is linked to several lifestyle and reproductive factors:

Delayed childbirth and lower rates of breastfeeding are associated with higher risks of certain cancers, including breast cancer. Rising obesity rates, decreased physical activity, and increased alcohol consumption contribute to the heightened cancer risk.

In 1943, the theory that the eventual cure for cancer would evolve from chemicals was not new. Dr. Charles Huggins, a University of Chicago urologist, concluded that the growth of cancer of the prostate gland upon the male hormone. If correct, he deduced that cancer could be controlled through the use of the female hormone. After receiving permission to castrate a patient dying of prostate cancer, he treated the dying man with the female hormone estrogen. The cancer was controlled, and the patient lived comfortably for the next fifteen years. This experience by Huggins proved that *the use of chemicals could definitely control some cancers* [emphasis added].

Despite the headwinds he was facing, Alexander continued his research into the reasons for the deaths at Bari.

In the initial paragraph of Alexander's preliminary report, he wrote, "The facts of [this report] are related as of December 17, at which time many of the detailed data, and especially the histopathology, are not available. Many of the observations in this report are based upon statements made by casualties or by medical officers and nurses who attended the cases, and only later study of the case records and data analysis will permit accurate appraisal and evaluation."

The report was widely distributed and scrutinized, particularly among medical facilities in the United States and Great Britain. It had a snowball effect on the medical population.

One officer was especially interested in the report: Col. Cornelius P. "Dusty" Rhoads, chief, Medical Division, Chemical Warfare Services. Rhoads was well-known throughout civilian and military medical circles, not only because he was commander of the Chemical Warfare Services but also because he was the head of New York City's large Memorial Hospital. Rhoads, often described as a "dynamo," had a profound fascination with conquering cancer, an obsession.

When he heard about the Bari bombing and the subsequent poisoning, he immediately decided to pursue an investigation into the matter—particularly after he read Col. Alexander's preliminary report; he sent the following to Alexander:

1. In connection with the slides of pathological specimens taken from casualties of the Bari incident, this office would appreciate being sent individual case reports so that the slides may be coordinated with individual cases.
2. Your cooperation in furnishing the previous report and sides is greatly appreciated. It is felt that the report and slides make a distinct contribution to the medical aspects of the agent concerned.

On 20 June 1944, Alexander fulfilled Rhoad's request and sent him his completed "Final Report of the Bari Mustard Casualties."

Most interesting, the letter that accompanied the report stated, "that medical observations concerning an explanation of why the case histories complied in the British hospital did not mention the chemical agent [mustard gas] but used the term 'NYD Dermatitis.'"

This was a reference by Alexander and others that what kept the matter suppressed was a command decision ordered by Winston Churchill in his quest to keep the matter top secret.

Rhoads carried his enthusiasm with him and returned to Memorial Hospital in New York City. All were convinced that chemicals could, indeed, be used to kill cancer but would leave normal cells alone.

Rhoads' excitement motivated and enthused others. He got the support of the vice president of Standard Oil, Alfred Sloan, who donated four million dollars, which started the construction of the soon-to-be-world-famous Sloan-Kettering Institute—the first institute in the world devoted only to cancer research. Dr. Rhoads continued directing the research at Sloan-Kettering until he died in 1959. Other important work continued: experimenting, testing, and developing nitrogen mustard compounds.

Dr. Gordon D. Jack, a surgeon, and colleagues worked for many years with the highly poisonous family of hydrogen mustard, especially in the field of lung cancer. If Jack had not interceded, 43 lung cancer patients would have perished within a month. Instead, Jack injected them with two large doses of tretamines, a nitrogen mustard drug. Ten of the cases experienced a marked to complete regression of the tumors. Three died within twelve days of the treatment, not of cancer, but from hemorrhaging from tumor masses that had been ravaged. The other seven survived, and four, the X-rays of the cancerous lungs returned to normal or nearly normal. Dr. Jack reported this in 1966 and the experiments continue today.

In 1961, headwinds persisted in the progress of discovering more about poisonous gas. That year, the Follow-Up Agency of the Division of Medical Sciences, National Academy of Sciences, National Research Council, Washington, D. C., began to study the physical condition of the Bari survivors—obstacles were aplenty—even for this highly prestigious organization. Trying to make headway, they almost always came up agains the "military secret" issue. Edgewood Arsenal, for example, "couldn't find" the complete records of the incident; the British records "were not available"; and few military officials knew or would admit that there even had been mustard at Bari—despite massive, irrefutable evidence. Eighteen years passed and almost all military people were still abiding Churchill's staunch desire to maintain mustard gas at Bari a military secret. And, too, the Director of the Follow-Up Agency was "undecided" how to approach the survivors about their health—that is, if they could be located, in itself a massive undertaking. The director approached Alexander asking, "Should we frame our approach in terms of the Bari disaster or conceal our underlying interest in a general study if the subsequent health of men who served overseas in World War II?" What Jack was really asking was should we or should we not tell the survivors that they had been exposed to mustard at Bari on 2 Dec. 1943? This was a monumental question that could conceivably open a can of worms. Imagine this happening today (2023)? The lawsuits would be massive. Damned if you do, damned if you don't.

Many of the survivors had no idea that there was poison gas in the Bari harbor that night or their affliction at the time was caused by mustard.

The United States Food and Drug Administration, in 1949, approved mechlorethamine, a nitrogen mustard compound—the first chemotherapy drug for hematologic malignancies. Then, about this time, scientists began to understand how the agent works in the body. Two chemists, Philip Lawley and Peter Brookes at the Royal Cancer Hospital, untangled the molecular mechanisms behind the agent's cancer-killing properties.

* * *

Despite a carapace of secrecy surrounding the incident at Bari, do we know how many people perished? How many people gave their lives for a medical breakthrough?

There is no accurate count.

However, it has been estimated that 1,000 men were killed

THE FATHER OF CHEMOTHERAPY

or went missing after the disaster—these, mostly seamen from American, British and private carriers. And after war's end, the years following the terrible incident, how many perished?

More than 800 were hospitalized. Of the casualties, about 628 suffered from mustard exposure.

After several hours, most patients appeared in good condition and were allowed to be sent to the Auxiliary Seaman's Home but clothed in oil contaminated clothing. They soon succumbed to the effects of the mustard.

How many Italian civilians suffered the same fate as military people is estimated to be around 1,000.

Safe to say about 2,000 died after the Germans left the harbor in acute pain.

Did Winston Churchill's command decision to keep the Bari incident a secret cause more deaths than necessary? Anyone familiar with warfare knows that there are many occasions when the few have to be sacrificed for the many. Churchill knew, too, that revealing what happened at Bari would most certainly have escalated the war and, overall, cause more deaths than those at Bari on 2 Dec.

Does humanity ever learn its lesson?

Apparently not.

Beginning in 2012, there were numerous reports of chemical weapons attacks in the Syrian Civil War. The attacks occurred in various areas of Syria, ordered by the recently deposed 23-year president Bashar al-Assad. The deadliest attacks were the August 2013 sarin attack in Ghouta (killing approximately 1,729 people and injuring 3,600, the April 2017 sarin attack in Khan Shaykhun (killing at least 89 people) and the April 2018 Douma chemical attacks (killing 43 people and injuring 500 civilians). The most common agent of choice used was chlorine. Between 2014 and 2018, a quarter of the attacks were delivered from the ground, half from aircraft, and the balance an indetermined method of delivery. Since the start of uprisings across Syria in 2011, Syrian Arab Armed Forces and pro-Assad paramilitary forces have been implicated in more than 300 chemical attacks in Syria.

In Syria, between October 2012 and May 2020, chemical attacks had been delivered on an almost monthly basis.

On 16 Dec. 2024, a bomb killed Russian General Igor Kirillov, 54, who died after an explosive device planted in a motor scooter was detonated near the entryway he had just exited of a residential building in Moscow. He was the highest-ranking military official killed inside Russia. The general was the chief of Russia's radioactive, chemical and biological defense forces. A day before his assassination, the Ukraine Security Service of Ukraine (SBU), the main law enforcement and security agency in Ukraine, responsible for counterintelligence, counterterrorism, national security, and state secrets protection, had charged General Kirillov in absentia, saying "he was responsible for the 'massive use of banned chemical weapons in Ukraine.'" The U.S. State Department said, "this spring Russia had used chloropicrin, a choking agent widely used in World War I, as well as tear gas on the battlefield. The Organization for the Prohibition of Chemical Weapons in May called the situation in Ukraine "volatile and extremely concerning regarding the possible re-emergence of use of toxic chemicals as weapons."

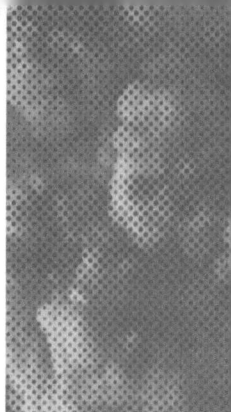

13

BARI

While the destruction of the port disrupted the flow of supplies to the Allied frontlines in Italy, it did not entirely stop the resupply effort. However, it did seriously hinder Doolittle's 15th Air Force bombing efforts in Europe, much to the relief of Kesselring—he had to know with certainty that the 15th would eventually get its wings back and resume its bombing of European cities, eventually forcing the surrender of the Third Reich.

Simultaneously, and according to Wolfram von Richtofen's plan, the success of the surprise air raid boosted German morale and demonstrated, albeit temporarily, the Luftwaffe's ability to continue the battle with its former strength. The accidental spread of the mustard gas was a bonus for the German's propaganda. The snake continued to squirm.

For Bari and the Allies, rebuilding the harbor and the surrounding areas of the city would take months, straining local and Allied resources. The destruction worsened an already difficult conditions for the local population, many of whom were displaced or faced shortages of essential goods, not the least of which was food. They would have to face the daunting reconstruction of their city, while at the same time deal with the challenges the war bought to their community. A intimidating task indeed, but one the citizens of Bari had shown through the centuries.

The best and perhaps most accurate description of Bari after the bombing of 2 December comes from our guide Lt. Henry Lowenhaupt.

Henry arrived in Bari on official duty in early March 1944, reporting to General Doolittle's Advanced Allied Air Force Headquarters, AKA the 15th Air Force Headquarters. How do we know with certainty Henry visited Bari months after the bombing, particularly after keeping silent about specific military details whatsoever? Here, in his letter of 5 March 1944, Henry clearly tells us that he has been assigned to Doolittle's headquarters in Bari. The organization was established at the Palazzo dell'Aeronautica, a building in Bari that served as a central administrative hub. While Henry mentions this fact, he makes no mention of military matters whatsoever.

After his arrival on 5 March 1944, Henry sat down and conveyed to paper his first impressions:

> I am writing for a moment while I am in an unsettled state. I am now in a hotel – where I may stay and may not – being presently assigned to the 15th Air Force Service Command – shall learn

possibly something of my status this afternoon. Until I do, I shall not write my new address.

What a drive I had yesterday – first – the driver formerly drove a New York taxi! Wheee! But it was magnificent – an all-day drive – through plains, over the mountains – magnificent country – and drive here, into fine, fertile, level country again. Fruit trees are in bloom – how Spring has sneaked up on me – and here there are fine, concrete roads, cities appearing to the eye undamaged. And such fine cities! This one (I have not seen much – it is Sunday, and places are closed) had, along the waterfront, heavy, fine buildings – magnificent, as Washington -

And such fine cities! This one [Bari](I have not seen much – it is Sunday, and places are closed) had, along the waterfront, heavy, fine buildings – magnificent, as Washington.

I walked through the new town, too, which is largely government or public buildings all along the waterfront – like an enormous WPA project. Shops all closed and nothing much for sale. I rested while getting a shampoo."

I am in a very beautiful place – a city substantially undamaged – fine buildings, lovely cathedral – an old walled town – the new section outside the walls – with beautiful surroundings – combination Atlanta City, St. Malo, Washington and Algiers – I think I should like to stay here – but don't care if I go elsewhere. My address is now [word unclear].

It is a cosmopolitan city – I was asking directions last night – the first man spoke only Yugoslavian – the next was an Indian who did not speak English – then an Italian who did not know – then a Scotsman, who did not know, and whom I couldn't understand anyway. Finally an American who knew.

I wish I could describe the magnificence of the drive yesterday – and the excitement of being in a city for a while. But I can't possibly – and feel that it won't last.

I am never going to write for anything again (I resolve, believing I shall break the resolution) for now I have things on the way I cannot possibly use. Well – I hate waste – but I shall nevertheless take the bull by the horns and throw stuff away. Blankets – woolen underwear – wool suits – alas! I am so overstocked!

I am well – curious as to what happens next. I am not sure I want to stay permanently in one place – it is bound to become boring, and in a city, there are many problems – as laundry, etc. pressing, and so forth. But I shall see what happens. I'm sure I don't know what I want.

All my love,
Henry

The Bari between 1944 and 1945 that Henry saw and ably described was a different city from the one seen today. It was already the second largest urban center in southern Italy (after

Naples, excluding the islands), with a population of about 200,000. The extent of the urban center was also limited to the Old Town, the nineteenth-century center (Murat), and the neighborhoods to the east (Umbertino, Madonnella, and monumental waterfront built during the Fascist period) and west (Libertà).

Bari Vecchia (Old Bari) is the historic heart of the city, located in the southern Italian region of Puglia (Apulia). It is the oldest part of the city and sits on a peninsula between two harbors, offering a glimpse into Bari's rich past, with narrow winding streets, ancient architecture, and a deeply rooted sense of history and tradition; it occupies a triangle of land jutting out into the sea. Many of the merchant ships waiting to be victims of the Luftwaffe were lined up along the moles here. A ferry terminal monopolizes the western side with two levels of seafront promenade on the eastern edge. One of these levels is the old walls, which, until the early 1900s, directly overlooked the sea. But by the 1940s, the lower level, the promenade that today runs along the peninsula, had already been built. As with most medieval towns, there's no pattern to the streets—all ziggy-saggy—but the district isn't big enough to get lost in for long.

It has long been one of the most popular and populated areas of the city, as

>beautiful as it is dangerous.

A gradual revaluation that began in the 2000s took the old town from a fiefdom of crime to a place of, first, nightlife and then massive tourism.

Today, the narrow streets are saturated with BnBs (Bed and Breakfasts), but you can still breathe the air of authenticity that characterizes Bari today.

Again, Henry, through keen eye, pen (or typewriter), and paper, presents us with a medley of grandeur and a travelogue's precise glimpse of this part of Bari.

Henry, on 6 March, continues imparting his experiences and impressions of Bari:

> My day today has been so mixed between military matters, about which as a matter of policy, I do not usually write, and non-military, that it is difficult to write. But I shall try to begin chronologically. As you know, I am now assigned to Air Corps – although I am still in Adjutant General Department. Yesterday, I reported to 15th AFSC and was told to come back this morning between 8 and 8:30, since the personnel officer was not there. So I went back – he was sick, but they would see him, and I should come back again at 1:30. He is the one to whom a cable was sent, saying that there was a vacancy for Clark and me elsewhere – did he need us urgently – and he replied "yes." But this is conventional, I suppose.
>
> So we walked up to the headquarters of 15th AAF, along the sea wall – and called on Major Staley – whom daddy knows – and talked for about an hour – he was quite cordial. Then we visited the adjutant general of 15th AAF [Major Gen Nathan F. Twining], and had lunch here at the hotel (Food is uninteresting – only messes are available)
>
> Then back to 15th AFSC – where they still did not know anything – and the personnel officer was displeased, he said, that we had let it be known we were here – But that does not disturb

me – he just wants to be sure that he controls our assignment – I do not care if he does not. Come back tomorrow -

So I spent the afternoon walking, especially through the old, walled town [Bari Vecchia], which is completely charming – archways, close streets, or alleys, squares, crowds – people cooking on the streets – colors (in which Italy excels) and a magnificent cathedral – St. Nicholas – without carvings and statues – a cloister. All the windows have been taken out – I hope for safekeeping.

Then, after wandering through the old city – which is endlessly intriguing, with its archways, its narrow passages, and howling of babies, women calling, all kinds of noises and smells, its carpenter shops, nuns, priests, all pushing through – I decided to have lunch on the hoof. A delicious orange, at the market, some candy, a cream puff, and, as always, I tried something that looked like chocolate cake but turned out to be figs and dates. [6 March]

Along Corso Cavour, one of the principal streets of Bari, Henry absorbs the beautiful thoroughfare, his mind certainly a camera clicking this and that for later recall with fingers later clicking at the office typewriter. Here's what he wrote of his self-guided tour:

This town[Bari] looks somewhat souvenir-less. It is too modern – the new part overwhelms the old – and no one seems to be attempting to capitalize on the willingness of soldiers to buy anything. All I have seen are souvenir picture postcards – which I cannot send because they would bare [V-Mail would prohibit this] the location in which I find myself (it is around you are familiar with all landscape and buildings!). [11 March]

First I walked across the railroad tracks – did not get beyond the town – and over there is the factory district, the warehouses (agricultural – figs, dates and so forth) I walked around a while – then bought a bottle of brandy and a bottle of Anisette. And walked back with them. It was beginning to rain, but the sidewalk had a double row of citron trees – which cover it close. I left my bottles here and went out on a double quest – not too determinedly. First, I stopped and got a haircut and shave. Then I went to a music store and asked a recommendation of a piano teacher. They gave me a name and address. I had to look for it a while – first asked a man who showed me the direction. Then, after a while that way, a woman, who must have thought she was a beauty. She tossed her head into the air and ran. Then I came upon it – and rang the bell. No answer." [14 march]

I enjoy walking in this town[Bari]. There is a main street [Corso Cavour] – six or eight blocks long, running from a corner of the old town and the sea – with a boulevard – and on the sidewalks double rows of trees which I think are lemon trees. Then in the boulevard larger trees. This is lined with fine buildings. Another main street [Corso Vittorio Emanuele] runs along the land side of the old town, at right angles to the first, and then drives along the shore, around the old city. The streets are heavily travelled with army trucks – But today, they were quite crowded with carriages – which are of all kinds. Many for hire – serve as taxis – then apparently many privately owned. Light little ones, the formal black ones – driving along the sea. And quite pretty horses. It makes the drive look much like a painting of the French painter whose name I've long tried to recall, who painted in spots. [19 March]

People dress up on Sunday and take walks – and it makes the sea-side walk look stylish and haute monde-ish with ladies and men and children all strolling along. Quite interesting – that is the new city. I haven't been in the old town on Sunday. [19 March]

Unquestionably, Henry enjoys his walks, and thanks to them we get an accurate glimpse of Bari after the bombing from a letter on 28 March:

I left the room shortly after seven – a windy morning, and ate breakfast – tomato juice, cereal, eggs, bacon, toast and coffee. Then walked out across the railroad tracks, and out of town – The day meanwhile having become cloudy. magnificent! A farm road, between high stone walls, over which the olive trees and fruit trees crowded. Here and there, open to a field – or through an open fence to a villa –as the Re David Villano – which is a great house, in a grove of pines, with formal, paved gardens, statuary of cupids and gods – the Italians work with stone so naturally that the garden statuettes even are handsome. Then the almond trees in bloom – and the petals blooming, like snow – the gentlest fragrance! Peasants plowing – carts going to town with artichokes and the like – quite fine horses – and gentlemen driving in carriages. Children running along the road in wooden shoes, strapped on, one carrying a flask of milk – looked like goat's milk. [28 March]

I am enjoying now the very beautiful, long evenings, which I usually spend walking, sometimes along the sea – which is, curiously, and without intended humor, called "The Board Walk." It is not board, but a wide street, without a sidewalk and a concrete balustrade along the sea. And into the old town, again, last night, where the streets were jam-packed with people going into and coming out of the churches, of which there must be seven or eight. The weather is now fine, although I note that it is clouding up a bit – for Tuesday, no doubt, my day off." [8 April]

I can have a very interesting time in this provincial town - which is completely magnificent to look at, too. I never get over the beauty of the old town – more lovely and exciting to me that the splendor of broad streets and formal statuary. But I like fine buildings, of which there are only a few here – the castle, the fortifications, the churches. The modern churches surpass my understanding. With the models of St. Nicholas and St. Theresa and other just a few blocks away, they build in the new town yellow brick or stone things just like suburban Chicago. [18 June]

Beyond the immediate damage caused by the air raid on 2 Dec., other parts of Bari suffered from sporadic bombings and military action throughout the balance of the war. The port area and nearby civilian districts were hardest hit, and the city underwent significant reconstruction in the post-war period. However, much of Bari's historic old town would survive the war intact. Meanwhile…

After an exploratory walking trip through Bari, Henry Lowenhaupt wrote another letter home. Here, he gives another accurate portrait of Bari:

> I enjoy walking in this town [Bari]. There is a main street [Corso Cavour was not the main street] – six or eight blocks long, running from a corner of the old town and the sea – with a boulevard – and on the sidewalks double rows of trees which I think are lemon trees. Then in the boulevard larger trees. This is lined with fine buildings. Another main street [Corso Vittorio Emanuele] runs along the land side of the old town, at right angles to the first, and then drives along the shore, around the old city. The streets are heavily travelled with army trucks – But today, they were quite crowded with carriages – which are of all kinds. Many for hire – serve as taxis – then apparently many privately owned. Light little ones, the formal black ones – driving along the sea. And quite pretty horses. It makes the drive look much like a painting of the French painter whose name I've long tried to recall, who painted in spots [he might be referring to Georges Seurat, who developed a style called Pointillism].

In a letter home sometime after the bombing, Henry describes the vecchia:

> The old town was as beautiful as ever. One place was selling hemp (I think it was that) and everywhere, old women had

gotten out their spindles and distaffs – and were spinning thread – quite a pretty process, although it is a very slow way of making thread. A spinning wheel is a modern, efficient method by comparison. They attach a little of the stuff to a bobbin, give the bobbin a whirl, and it spins and twists a thread. Then they wind the thread on the bobbin, and spin it again, making more. I have not seen any weaving here.

The charm here rested in the narrow, winding streets with a labyrinth of alleyways, roads, and squares. Many of them filled with historical sites such as the Arch of Marvels, Basilica of San Nicola (Santa Claus), Pizza Ferrarse, and Largo San Pietro.

Then, on 14 and 15 May, Henry could not resist a visit to Santa Clause's burial site, the Basilica of San Nicola:

So I walked a while. I went to church, and through it. It is not one of the finest examples – that is, not up to Morreale [France] and Rouen and Notre Dame de Paris – but it is lovely – the tomb of St. Nicholas, they say, in cast silver, which I don't fully appreciate. Beautiful stairway on the tomb of the Queen of Poland. Beautiful columns, shape – one misses the color of stained-glass windows – but I suppose it may be these southern churches never had them."

Today being my day off, I have done intensive loafing all day – walking through the town, old and new, looking in ship windows, watching children and what not, with my music lesson at noon – which is still the high point of my week. I enjoy it very much, I went into the cathedral - I do not find it as inspiring or as beautiful as I expect – maybe because I do not understand this conservative, solid architecture – and am come to expect vaults and gothic windows. Still, it is unquestionably a solid piece of stone building, with many delicate details of stone carving. The tomb itself – a great piece of silver, with scenes from the life of the saint I cannot understand at all as a thing of beauty.

But I believe it is generally fine that beautiful Italian things are usually much less striking than French or Greek – and I have come to think of fine Italians as much more conservative than the English even, and with feeling very deep – and self-contained. Not at all like Spanish or others, with superficial decoration. I believe it may take quite a little time for the merit of a thing like this cathedral to grow on you. It is enormously quiet and heavy and dignified – very little color – but that there is (some ceiling paintings and a few others) very modern in its contrast and the natural color is everywhere so high, that the old gray green of the stone is restful. It is so completely far from tawdry and decorated. I think the more often I go there, the more I shall enjoy it.

The same is true of the whole old town – the walls, the old castle – heavy and plain – but they grow very interesting as you watch them, and very dignified – way beyond the dignity of the inhabitants and naked pa babies squawking in the streets. I come to think from this especially that fine Italian people are something superfine – but most you see are poor, dirty beggars.

While Bari did not experience destruction, the city suffered substantial damage, particularly to its port and the immediate areas adjacent to the bombed harbor.

During a visit while this book was being written, Charles Lowenhaupt, Henry's father visited Bari and retraced some of his father's footsteps. This is a portion of what he wrote:

> If you look at a map of Bari you can see that the peninsula of the old town separates the harbor bombed from the old harbor and most of the Fascist Bari that father [Henry] would have seen his first day. We believe that his apartment was in the new part of town back from Lungomare [a lungormare is a boardwalk]. The university, train tracks, and everything else he would have seen the first day (including headquarters of Air Force0 is separated from the bombed harbor by the old city and the Castle. This was very clear as we walked around Bari this month. So was the University where he went to the library, and even his piano teacher's house was just inside old town but on the South side. So much of what he would have seen was apparently not damaged by the bombing or if damaged only some broken glass. Today the harbor that was bombed is a kind of fortress requiring special passes or a plan on a ferry to get in (though our guide got us in by explaining that my father had been in the army during the time period. It is today a bustling harbor with ferries and cruise ships. The charming little harbor with fishermen selling their shellfish every morning is completely removed and protected by the old town from the big harbor.

Sometime after the war, General Doolittle retired and moved to St. Louis and lived in the same Parkview neighborhood that Henry's grandparents lived in. Parkview was one of the early "suburban" creations in the United States. Henry's parents were known in the neighborhood for having a cow which escaped one rainy day and ruined the neighbor's yards. Because he worked for Doolittle at the 15th Air Force Headquarters, Henry had to have known about the Bari bombing but never mentioned it in any of his letters home.

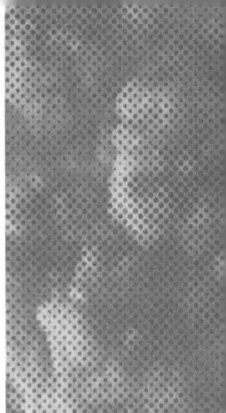

CODA

On 2 May 1945, *Generalfeldmarschall* Albert "Smilin' Al" Kesselring convened a meeting of his commanders in Austria and neighboring regions. The subject was how to best protect his men after the Germans surrendered. Numerous plans were crafted to effect this so that others could retreat—an act on the field marshal's part to save as many of his men as possible. At this time, the German government was establishing peace terms with the Allies, which limited how much time Kesselring had to safely get his men away from capture by the Red Army.

However, none of these and other Kesselring qualities eclipsed the fact that, after war's end, Kesselring was convicted as a war criminal for his involvement and responsibility for several war crimes committed under his flag during World War II. Specifically, the massacres of civilians, including the infamous Ardeatine Cave massacre in outside of Rome in March 1944. There, 335 Italian civilians were executed in the Ardeatine Caves by the SS under the command of *SS-Obersturmbannführers* (Lieutenant Colonel) Herbert Kappler, a reprisal for an Italian partisan attack that killed 33 *Ordnungspolizei* (Order Police, "Orpo") on Via Rasella, a narrow residential street in Rome.

In 1947, after the war, Kesselring was tried by a British military court. He was found guilty of war crimes, specifically the mass murder of civilians in connection with the aforementioned massacres and reprisals. Initially sentenced to death by hanging (a dishonorable execution for a German officer, as opposed to a firing squad). However, his sentence was later commuted to life imprisonment because of his popularity with influential Allied politicians and generals. This was partly due to various factors, including political considerations during the early Cold War period and appeals from German and Italian veterans' groups. He was released from prison in 1952 on grounds of ill health. On 16 July 1960, Albert Kesselring died of a heart attack. Hundreds of veterans attended his funeral, remembering him fondly. However, he remained a contentious figure, beloved by his former troops, but rejected by a German establishment that was striving to forget its past actions in Italy, looking at them as unforgiveable and murderous. In the end, Kesselring was an effective leader but nevertheless a convicted war criminal.

Generalfeldmarschall Wolfram von Richtofen often looked upon similarly to Kesselering as an effective leader and innovator but nevertheless a war criminal because of the aerial bombings he ordered in Guernica in 1937 and Warsaw in 1939. The sensationalistic press coverage of these and other events included "grossly inflated casualty figures" that did not help von Richtofen's legacy. Von Richtofen issued contracts that led to the development of the first practical cruise missile, the V-1, and the first long-range ballistic missile. His biographer states that he can be seen as "one of air powers visionaries." Throughout 1944 he suffered from headaches and exhaustion due to a brain tumor. He passed away on 12 July 1945 as an American prisoner of war. Ironically, he died in a United States Air Force hospital in Bad Ischl, Austria.

After the war, *Oberstleutnant* (Lieutenant Colonel) Werner Baumbach, the German officer with the Hollywood movie star looks, was imprisoned for three years; he subsequently moved to Argentina and began work as a test pilot. On 20 Oct. 1953, age of thirty-six, while evaluating a British Lancaster bomber for the Argentine Air Force, Baumbach died when the plane he was testing crashed near Berazategui, Argentina. He was interred in his hometown, Kloppenburg, Lower Saxony, Germany. The street *Werner-Baumbach-Straßein* was named after him.

British Air Marshal Sir Arthur "Mary" Coningham, after 30 years of exemplary commissioned service, retired from the Royal Air Force. On 30 Jan. 1948 he vanished when the airliner on which he was traveling to Bermuda disappeared off the east coast of Florida. Nary a trace was found of the aircraft or Coningham.

When the war ended Dr. Stewart F. Alexander returned to Park Ridge, New Jersey and established a distinguished medical career. He became the medical director of Bergen Pines County Hospital (now known as New Bridge Medical Center) until 1975. He was also an active internist and cardiologist, and held numerous leadership positions, including president of the Bergen County Medical Society.

After receiving an honorable discharge from the Army on Christmas day 1945, Captain Henry Cronbach Lowenhaupt, our astute letter writer, returned to St. Louis, where he began practicing a distinguished career in law. We wonder if Henry ever visited with General Doolittle while in St. Louis.

Between 1948 and 1950, Henry served as the Excess Profits Tax Counsel in Washington, D.C. He was a founder of Temple Emanuel in St. Louis and served on the board of the Community School in St. Louis. Most notable, he argued a number of important cases in the US Supreme Court, including International Shoe vs. the State of Washington. Many of his court cases are considered quite impactful, most famously one of his arguments3 stated that the US Tax Court was unconstitutional as it was reconstructed in 1969. Henry continued to play piano throughout his life. In his 60's, he started tying "oriental rugs" one knot at a time. He spent most weekends at a country house in Silex, Missouri, where he tied rugs and read voraciously. Henry Cronbach Lowenhaupt died on October 24, 1990.

Little is known about the path Hauptmann Veit Renz's life took after war's end. It has not been determined if he received the *Ehrenpokal der Luftwaffe*, the Luftwaffe silver Honor Goblet he hoped for after completing his five reconnaissance missions of Bari's harbor.

* * *

Days, weeks and months after the bombing, Bari's citizens as well as the Allied forces went to work repairing the harbor and the city. All had a job—win the war and push the Germans out of their country.

Throughout the period of writing this book, the author had numerous email exchanges with Henry's son, Charles. One in particular stands out, a lesson in the spirit of human strength and resilience. Through Henry's letters we experience the resolve of people living through a hopeless time but enduring—endurance often the substance of success. His letters mostly tell us, not about the battles of war, but the battles the Italian people had to endure to merely survive. Charles wrote the following:

> … It seems to me there is a lesson in my father's letters and that is the resilience of the human-Italian character. In fact after all the devastation, within 3 months there is a return to normalcy that allows Henry to write home without reference to the devastation and depict a city (yes a city) returning to cultural and human normalcy—operas, dinners, a trip to Rome as a holiday, etc. There is so much that can be seen here. I must say that personally after I read all the horror of that attack and what followed and the heroism of Alexander and others, I am even more moved by the letters and what they reflect. And more moved by Bari and my own visit there. It is no Hiroshima or Berlin or any other city destroyed in the war. It rebuilt and with character over the subsequent months.

Special gratitude goes to Charles A. Lowenhaupt for providing his father's letters and a collection of invaluable details in a historic story involving a momentous and partially forgotten event during World War II. The bombing and subsequent destruction and suffering was an event that was also a starting point for discovering the benefits of chemotherapy.

* * *

On 20 May 1988, US Army historians held a small ceremony in Washington. There, a white-haired Stewart Alexander, former US Army colonel, received a long over-do military honor. Several senators where present, pleased to give Alexander his due. After all, his efforts had an enormous impact that pressed beyond his patients—those efforts became a "catalyst for developing chemotherapy." Alexander was presented with a Certification of Appreciation signed by the Army surgeon general. It read: "Without his early diagnosis and rapid initiation of appropriate and aggressive treatment, many more lives would have been lost and the severity of injuries would have been much greater. His service to the military and civilians injured during the catastrophe reflects the finest measure of a soldier and physician."

Oddly and refreshingly, Captain Mark Yow, assistant officer to the surgeon general, spoke some truth at the ceremony, saying that US Army "could not have honored Alexander until recently, when the British declassified the documents relating to the incident."

Alexander, maintaining his humility, said, "This [award] is not something I ever sought. I did what I saw as my duty at the time, as I always have all my life."

Alexander also said he thought Churchill's command decision was the right one, adding that Churchill was one of his "political heroes." But, adding, "I think he was unduly harsh in his management of it."

The story of Alexander's investigation into the Bari incident, and the Army Surgeon General's award, were read into the Congressional Record.

While packing for a Thanksgiving vacation in the Caribbean with his daughter and three grandchildren, Alexander took a phone call from London: the British government wanted to present him with high honors for his work in Bari. "I'm sorry," he said, "but after so many years it will have to wait a little longer. I'm leaving on holiday and will have to discuss the matter upon my return."

This was a poignant moment.

Because Alexander knew then he would not live to receive his honors.

On 6 Dec. 1991, aged seventy-seven, Steward Alexander died.

He knew what the cause of his death would be—he had diagnosed himself.

Malignant melanoma—skin cancer.

The Army Surgeon General's award and the full story of Bari were read into the Congressional Record. Even Alexander's *The New York Times* obituary kept Bari out of the news—it made no mention of the Bari bombing or mustard gas, and not a word about chemotherapy.

That fall in 1988, Representative Margaret "Marge" Roukema of New Jersey, paid the highest tribute she could calling Alexander "The Father of Chemotherapy."

Alexander's efforts and the deaths and agony of hundreds of service people and the citizens of Bari on 2 Dec., was a key step toward decreasing the pain and suffering of countless patients since that fateful night and furthering the effort to abolish cancer once and for all.

Many shall always be grateful.

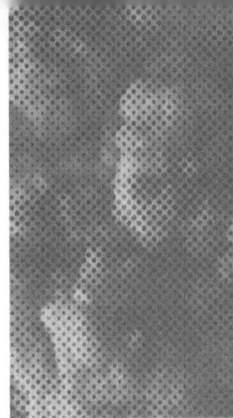

BIBLIOGRAPHY

Bender, R. J. (1972). Air Organizations of the Third Reich: The Luftwaffe. Palo Alto: D-D Associates.

Conant, J. (2020). The Great Secret: The Classified World War II Disaster that Launched the War On Cancer. New York, NY: Norton.

Editors, C. R. (2020). Field Marshal Albert Kesselring: The Life and Legacy of Nazi Germany's Most Popular Commander. Charles River Editors.

Elphick, P. (2001). Liberty Ships: The Ships That Won the War. Annapolis, MD: Naval Institute.

Hamilton, C. (1996). Leaders & Personalities of the Third Reich, Their Biographies, Portraits and Autographs Volume 1. San Jose: R. James Bender Publishing.

Hamilton, C. (1996). Leaders & Personalities of the Third Reich, Their Biographies, Portraits and Autographs Volume 2. San Jose: R. James Bender Publishing. https://en.wikipedia.org/wiki/Air_Raid_on_Bari.

https://www.smithsonianmag.com/history/bombing-and-breakthrough-180975505/. (2020, Setpyember).

Infield, G. (2020). Disaster at Bari: The Terrifying World War II Chemical Warfare Castastrophe.

Lowenhaupt, Charles A. 2024. The War Letters of Henry C. Lowenhaupt
- 1943-1944. Estes Park: Armin Lear Press.

Reminick, G. (2001). Nightmare In Bari. Palo Alto: Glencannon Press.

Robert M. Browning, J. (1996). U.S. Merchant Vessel War Casualities of World
War II. Annapolis: Naval Instituted Press.

Periodicals and Letters

Henry C. Lowenhaupt Taped Interview, February 6, 1986

Bari During the Occupation

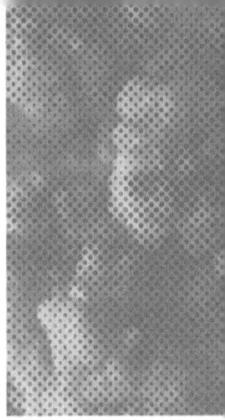

ABOUT THE AUTHOR

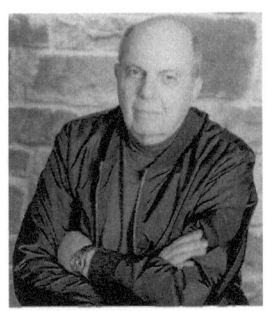

Vincent dePaul Lupiano is the author of three WWII military history books in addition to the *The WWII Bombing of Bari: Operation Tidal Wave—The Bloodiest Air Battle in the History of War*, *Operation Ginny—The Most Significant Commando Raid of WWII*, and *Massacre at Oradour-sur-Glane—Nazi Gold and the Murder of an Entire French Town by SS Division Das Reich*, with all three published by Lyons Press. He has published two novels under the pseudonym Christopher Sloan, *In Search of Eagles*, and *The Wings of Death*. His international political thrillers, *One Minute to Midnight* and *Deadlight* were published by Armin Lear Press.

He spent many years as program director, writer, and host of his radio program at WFAS in White Plains, NY. In New York City, he worked at WOR-TV and WOR-AM as a promotional writer and producer. At the American Broadcasting Company's WABC and WPLJ, he was a writer, producer, and editorial director. He also worked at IBM for ten years as a speechwriter to senior executives, editor of a management publication, producer, and director of corporate films and videos. He was born and raised in Manhattan, New York City, and currently resides in Franklin Lakes, NJ, with his dog, Chase.

www.ingramcontent.com/pod-product-compliance
Lightning Source LLC
Chambersburg PA
CBHW020052170426
43199CB00009B/257